CLINICAL PEDIATRIC ONCOLOGY

Research, Diagnosis, Treatment and Prognosis of Malignant Tumors of Childhood

CLINICAL PEDIATRIC ONCOLOGY

Research Diagnosis Treatment and Prognosis of Malignant Tumors of Childhood

Selected topics from the ANNUAL RADIOTHERAPY SYMPOSIUM sponsored by the Department of Radiation Oncology, Cedars of Lebanon Health Center and the Department of Pediatrics, University of Miami School of Medicine, Miami, Florida.

Edited by

MARIO M. VUKSANOVIC, M.D.

A *Symposia Specialists* book

Published by

FUTURA PUBLISHING COMPANY, INC.

Mount Kisco, New York 10549 U.S.A.

Library of Congress Catalog
Card Number 72-80549
ISBN 0-87993-009-8

Available from

FUTURA PUBLISHING COMPANY, INC.

295 Main Street
Mount Kisco, New York 10549

Contents

Introduction

The Fifth Annual Radiotherapy Symposium entitled "Clinical Pediatric Oncology" represents the garnering of knowledge and experience of the experts in the field of pediatric oncology. Cancer in children is the cause of twenty percent of all deaths under the age of fifteen and is second only to accidental deaths in this age category. In the last decade, cancer has become an increasingly important pediatric problem because prevention and effective treatment have coupled to reduce the threat of infection. It also appears that there has been an absolute increase in the incidence of cancer in children.

The management of the child with cancer differs considerably from the care of the adult with cancer and the problems vary with the age of the child. These problems include variations in the awareness and understanding of the illness by the child, the reaction of the parents to the child's illness, the effect on siblings in the family unit, and the impact on the child's development.

The papers presented in this volume demonstrate the need for the development of a multidiscipline approach to the care of the child with cancer. In institutions where such programs are well developed, the combined aggressive therapy utilizing surgery, radiation therapy, and chemotherapy has resulted, in almost every instance, with increased survival and improved quality of care. This is illustrated particularly in Wilm's tumor where the cure rate doubled in the last ten years. Also, significant and improved survival has resulted from combined management in patients with rhabdomyosarcoma, Ewing's sarcoma, neuroblastoma, and leukemia. In the latter case, the introduction of the total therapy approach to acute lymphocytic leukemia has been marked by a closely integrated program employing chemotherapy and radiation therapy with a marked and significant improvement in the survival from disease. There is now the possibility of a fifty percent five-year "cure" rate within reach of every child with acute lymphocytic leukemia.

The authors deal with the side effects from treatment and point out that the risk of complication must be considered within the perspective of survival.

Of great importance also is the physician's need to manage the problems in communication which frequently exist among the collaborating physicians, parents, and nursing staff in the care of the fatally ill child or adolescent. Failures in communication often reflect imperfect health care systems and hospital practices, inadequate attention to the psychological needs of the parent, little appreciation for the developmental aspects of the child's concept of death, and failure to recognize and support common coping mechanisms seen in both the child and his parents. This problem of communication in the care of fatally ill children is articulately and clearly expressed in the article by Dr. Stanford B. Friedman.

The symposium demonstrates the need for the development of multidiscipline teams skilled and trained in the care of the child with cancer, the employment of all the facilities at hand, including surgery, radiation therapy, and chemotherapy in order to achieve the maximum cure rate, as well as the optimum in quality of survival. In centers where multidiscipline teams exist, complications from treatment can be kept to a minimum and the standardization of treatment programs can be achieved. The child with cancer represents a national resource which should be utilized in national cooperative clinical trials to determine the most appropriate programs of management. Only by such trials will the definitive knowledge as to the most effective form of treatment by developed.

Dr. Vuksanovic and his colleagues are to be commended for the quality of the symposium and for its excellent scientific merit.

Luther W. Brady, M.D.
Professor and Chairman
Department of Radiation Therapy
and Nuclear Medicine
Hahnemann Medical College
and Hospital
Philadelphia, Pennsylvania

Foreword

Interest generated in malignancy in childhood is not merely a casual one. The awareness of its importance became quite obvious through statistical reporting from various sources, indicating that the mortality rate due to cancer in children under the age of 15 years is second only to accidents in this age group.

According to some workers, there has been apparently an absolute increase in the incidence of cancer in children in the last decade. Moreover, the kinds of malignant tumors and their biological behavior differ from the adult population affected by malignant neoplasia. Some kinds of cancer in childhood simply do not have their counterpart in adults.

The past decade has witnessed extraordinary development in the pediatric oncology. Both specialty as well as lay press abounds with optimistic initial reports of cures in previously unconquerable malignant diseases of children, such as acute leukemia. Along the same line, one cannot but become enthusiastic in receiving data which indicate possible cures in children with a perspective of survivalship of 50 or more years. For the same reason the enthusiasm generated by initial successes should have careful analysis of rapidly changing concepts and necessity of more prolonged follow-up.

In the Fifth Annual Radiotherapy Symposium an assembly of specialists and researchers interested in the field of childhood cancer have gathered to present and discuss a considerable acumen of scientific interest. Participants to the Symposium have repeatedly expressed their satisfaction, if not hope, in reports which demonstrate that we might indeed be on the threshold of spectacular importance in management of some of the childhood malignant tumors. No doubt the joint effort and exchange of information of basic researchers and clinicians of various specialties have borne this early promising fruit. Through combination of surgery, chemo, and radiation therapy and through better understanding of the biological behavior of childhood oncology these achievements have become possible. It is then in the multidisciplinary approach to the problem that some further improvements could be expected. We hope to share our enthusiasm generated by these proceedings through exchange of information in the volume that clearly demonstrates that awareness of oncological biology and need of application in clinical medicine by various specialists has become a common denominator to further successes.

Mario M. Vuksanovic

Acknowledgments

The Annual Radiotherapy Symposium on Pediatric Oncology expresses its sincere thanks to the following institutions for their support:

American Cancer Society, Florida Division, Inc.

Merck Sharp & Dohme

Florida Regional Medical Program
for Childhood Cancer

Varian Associates

Warm thanks are rendered to the Administration of Cedars of Lebanon Health Center, to the Board of Trustees, and to our voluntary faculty.

Mario M. Vuksanovic, M.D.
Chairman
Annual Radiotherapy Symposium

Peculiarities in the Occurrence of Childhood Cancer: Epidemiologic and Etiologic Considerations

Joseph F. Fraumeni, Jr., M.D.

Childhood cancer has traditionally been viewed as a sporadic, isolated, or random event. Only recently have systematic efforts been made to examine the disease in an epidemiologic context. The patterns of occurrence for childhood cancer reveal a number of peculiarities that provide clues to the etiology of this disease.

Demographic Patterns

Peculiarities in the distribution of childhood cancer in populations suggest risk factors in carcinogenesis, and are a valuable source of hypotheses that can be tested or evaluated by more definitive epidemiologic studies.

Age. A peak in mortality under five years of age occurs for many of the common cancers, such as leukemia, certain brain tumors, neuroblastoma, and Wilms's tumor.[1] For some cancers the peaks occur so early in life that a large proportion, if not all, must originate *in utero*.

Age curves for other tumors suggest postnatal influences. For example, bone cancer increases in frequency with age through childhood and adolescence, and closely resembles the age curves for skeletal growth, which may be a stimulus to the development of bone cancer.[1,2] Hodgkin's disease, rare under five years of age, has a slow climb in mortality, more pronounced in boys, until 11 years of age.[3,4] Then the rates for each sex rise sharply toward the first large peak around 25 to 30 years of age. The abrupt change in death rates at 11 years suggests an increased susceptibility or exposure to some agent three or more years earlier, since the average survival from childhood Hodgkin's disease is about 2-3 years.[3] The susceptibility has been linked to the spontaneous involution of lymphoid tissues that occurs during childhood,[3] a hypothesis consistent with a recently reported association between tonsillectomy and Hodgkin's disease.[5]

Joseph F. Fraumeni, Jr., M.D., *Head, Ecology Studies Section, Epidemiology Branch, National Cancer Institute, Bethesda, Maryland.*

Sex. Cancer is generally more common in boys than girls; an exception is teratoma, which predominates in girls.[6] The peak in early childhood is due primarily to teratomas of the pre-sacral region, whereas the rising frequency after six years results from gonadal tumors. Female preponderance at both sites suggests a common origin. For example, multi-potential germ cells appear to account for gonadal teratomas; and these cells, if trapped outside the developing gonad, may give rise to pre-sacral teratomas.[6]

Race. The towering peak for leukemia at four years of age in the U. S. occurs only for white children, with no trace of an increase among nonwhites.[1,7] The peak is specific for the acute lymphocytic type of leukemia. The myelogenous form shows little variation until adolescence, when both races show a small second peak. It has been suggested that prenatally or very soon after birth white children are affected by leukemogenic influences to which nonwhite children are either not susceptible or not exposed.[7] The small adolescent peak for myelogenous leukemia may be related to hormonal stimuli at the time of puberty.

Another example of racial variation was found recently in a mortality survey of bone tumors.[2] The frequencies of osteogenic sarcoma showed no difference by race, but Ewing's sarcoma was virtually absent among Negro children. This finding has etiologic implications, and is a clinical feature that should be considered whenever Ewing's tumor is entertained as a diagnosis in a Negro patient.

International differences. Certain tumors show marked geographic variation in risk which provides opportunities for studying environmental factors. For example, children in Africa are prone to Burkitt's lymphoma, Kaposi's sarcoma, and liver cancer,[8] in Brazil, to Hodgkin's disease, adrenocortical tumors, and renal carcinoma[9]; and in Jamaica, to retinoblastoma.[10]

High Risk Groups

Much has been learned recently by studies of persons who are exceptionally liable to develop childhood cancer.

Leukemia and lymphoma. Comprehensive information on leukemia has been assembled by Miller.[11] The highest risk occurs for identical twins of leukemic children, who have a 1 in 5 risk of leukemia, which develops within weeks or months after the disease is diagnosed in the co-twin. In patients with polycythemia vera treated with radiation, the risk is 1 in 6 that leukemia develops within 10 to 15 years. In Bloom's syndrome, and probably Fanconi's syndrome, the risk is about 1 in 8 that leukemia will occur under 30 years of age. Survivors of Hiroshima who were within 1000 meters of the atomic blast have a risk of 1 in 60 within 12 years of exposure. Children with Down's syndrome or mongolism have a risk of 1 in 95 before their 10th birthday. Patients with ankylosing spondylitis treated with radiation show a risk of 1 in 270 within 15 years of exposure. Siblings of leukemic children have a risk of 1 in 720. For comparison, one child in nearly 3000 in this country will develop the disease before the tenth birthday.

Common to these groups is a genetic or cytogenetic feature.[11] Identical twins are genetically identical, and sibs are genetically similar. Extra chromosomes have been reported with polycythemia vera before radiation therapy, and a characteristic extra chromosome in the the G-group occurs in Down's syndrome. Patients with the congenital syndromes of Bloom and Fanconi show chromosome fragility, and ionizing radiation can produce long-lasting chromosomal breaks.

Persons prone to leukemia are not at similar risk of lymphoma, which occurs excessively in persons with congenital immune-deficiency disorders, such as Wiskott-Aldrich syndrome, agammaglobulinemia, and ataxia-telangiectasia.[11-15] This epidemiologic distinction suggests that leukemia and lymphoma should be distinguished in etiologic investigations. The immune-deficiency disorders, however, do predispose to one type of leukemia, namely the acute lymphocytic variety.

Furthermore, the risk of leukemia and lymphoma is increased in conditions which are acquired after birth, and are accompanied by cytogenetic or immunologic abnormalities.[11-15] The agents which are known or suspected to cause leukemia – ionizing radiation, benzene, probably alkylating agents, and possibly chloramphenicol – also have the capacity to damage chromosomes and depress the bone marrow. The acquired conditions predisposing to lymphoma include Sjogren's syndrome and non-tropical sprue, but the most striking risk occurs among patients receiving immunosuppressive therapy with kidney transplants.

Wilms' tumor and other cancers. The complex of anomalies associated with leukemia and lymphoma are quite different from those related to Wilms' tumor,[16] neoplasms of the adrenal cortex,[17] and hepatoblastoma.[18] These conditions occur excessively in children who have various forms of congenital growth excess: hemihypertrophy, hamartomatous growths (including extensive nevi), and the visceral-cytomegaly syndrome.[12,19]

Another defect associated with Wilms' tumor, but not with other neoplasms, is congenital aniridia (bilateral absence of the iris). Children with this syndrome have a variety of non-ocular anomalies, such as craniofacial dysmorphism, recurved external ear, receding chin, and undescended testes.[20] Aniridia is extremely rare in the general population, but in children with Wilms' tumor the defect is about a thousand times greater than usual. In a multi-hospital series of 440 children with Wilms' tumor, 6 had aniridia.[16] Approaching the association in the opposite fashion, 27 young children were followed with aniridia, and

Wilms' tumor developed subsequently in 6.[20] Ordinarily aniridia is due to an autosomal dominant gene, and two-thirds of the cases have a family history of the defect. With Wilms' tumor, however, aniridia is nearly always non-familial, indicating that the eye defect and the tumor are due to a fresh gene mutation, or to an environmental agent that mimics the action of a gene.[12] Although both aniridia and hemihypertrophy predispose to Wilms' tumor, the two anomalies do not seem to occur together. Yet both anomalies and Wilms' tumor are linked with congenital defects of the genitourinary tract.[12] All pathways point to a developmental defect of the kidney, which should be clarified by further study of high-risk patients.

Thus, much can be learned about etiologic mechanisms by identifying constellations of diseases linked to cancer. The relationships found between teratogenesis and oncogenesis suggest that childhood cancer can be studied in terms of what is known about the origin of the associated malformation.[12] Furthermore, the careful follow-up of high-risk children may lead to the early diagnosis of cancer and life-saving surgery.

Familial Occurrence

Epidemiologic surveys have revealed that the siblings of children with certain cancers, such as leukemia and brain tumor, have a significantly increased risk of the same cancer.[21] Such occurrences, when observed clinically, may be used for etiologic study. For example, a battery of laboratory studies was applied to a family with an aggregation of acute myelogenous leukemia, affecting three children and three adults.[22] It had been shown previously that skin fibroblasts taken by biopsy from patients born with a high risk of leukemia, such as mongolism and Fanconi's syndrome, were extremely sensitive to transformation *in vitro* by the tumor virus, SV-40. This family showed high rates of fibroblast transformation among surviving patients and other family members on the line of descent. The study is an illustration of the value of high-risk groups in assessing newly developed indicators of cancer susceptibility.

Cancers of *different* sites or cell types may also occur excessively in the same family. For example, the siblings of children with brain tumor have an increased risk not only for brain tumor, but also for sarcomas of soft tissue and bone.[21] New syndromes may be detected also by studies of individual families. To illustrate this point, two young cousins were observed with rhabdomyosarcoma, and the family history revealed a striking concentration of breast cancer and other neoplasms in the pedigree.[23,24] This observation prompted a multi-hospital survey of rhabdomyosarcoma in children, and three patients were found to have a sibling with rhabdomyosarcoma. In all families, there was an increased frequency of other neoplasms, particularly breast cancer, in the parents and other young adults. Some members of these families had double primary tumors.

The familial multiple-cancer syndromes may be related to the phenomenon of multiple primary cancer in the same person. The tumors, rather than concentrating in one person, may be scattered over the family tree. Constellations of multiple cancer in individuals and in families suggest that these cancers have etiologic factors in common.

Prenatal Origins

Evidence accumulated by Miller[25] indicates that many childhood cancers are determined by events in prenatal life. For example, early age peaks for certain tumors suggest an origin before birth. Sometimes the cancers develop rapidly during intrauterine life, and are diagnosed at birth or soon after. The association between certain cancers and malformations indicates that both arise during embryonic development. Furthermore, the prenatal influence may be prezygotic; for example, genetic neoplasms like retinoblastoma, or preneoplastic states like neurofibromatosis, xeroderma pigmentosa, and the inherited syndromes associated with chromosome breakage or immune deficiency. The familial tendencies observed for the more common cancers of children appear to be determined at least partly by genetic susceptibility, but the precise mechanisms are far from clear. The high concordance rate for childhood leukemia in identical twins has been attributed to genetic factors, but may also be due to the transplantation of pre-leukemic stem cells from one twin to another through a shared placental circulation. An increased risk of all cancers has been reported among children exposed *in utero* to ionizing radiation. Such exposures can probably cause leukemia, as in postnatal irradiation at any age, but there is some doubt as to whether very low doses to the fetus will induce *all* forms of childhood cancer equally.[26]

Finally, prenatal factors may cause cancers which do not occur until after childhood. A few months ago, investigators from the Massachusetts General Hospital reported a cluster of eight young women in the Boston area with adenocarcinoma of the vagina, an uncommon disease usually restricted to the elderly.[27] The patients were between 14 and 22 years of age. A retrospective study revealed that the mothers of seven had been given stilbestrol during pregnancy to prevent miscarriage. In a matched control group of 32 mothers, none had been given the drug. Five additional young women with vaginal cancer were then discovered this past year through the New York State Tumor Registry, and all five mothers had received synthetic estrogens during pregnancy.[28] These remarkable observations indicate that transplacental carcinogenesis has occurred in man after a latent period of 14-22 years. Follow-up studies of women who were exposed *in utero* to synthetic estrogens are presently underway to enable early diagnosis and to clarify the extent of the cancer risk.

Conclusions

The epidemiologic patterns of childhood cancer show many peculiarities which should assist efforts in etiologic research, differential diagnosis, surveillance for the early detection and therapy of cancer, and the counseling of susceptible children and families.

References

1. Ederer, F., Miller, R. W. and Scotto, J.: U. S. childhood cancer mortality patterns, 1950-59. *JAMA* 192:593-596, 1965.
2. Glass, A. G. and Fraumeni, J. F., Jr.: Epidemiology of bone cancer in children. *J. Nat. Cancer Inst.* 44:187-199, 1970.
3. Miller, R. W.: Mortality in childhood Hodgkin's disease. *JAMA* 198:1216-1217, 1966.
4. Fraumeni, J. F., Jr. and Li, F. P.: Hodgkin's disease in childhood: an epidemiologic study. *J. Nat. Cancer Inst.* 42:681-691, 1969.
5. Vianna, N. J., Greenwald, P. and Davies, J. N. P.: Tonsillectomy and Hodgkin's disease: the lymphoid tissue barrier. *Lancet* 1:431-432, 1971.
6. Fraumeni, J. F., Jr. and Hill, N. A.: Mortality from malignant teratomas in childhood (Abstract). *Teratology* 2:260, 1969.
7. Court Brown, W. M. and Doll, R.: Leukemia in childhood and young adult life. *Brit. Med. J.* 1:981-988, 1961.
8. Davies, J. N. P.: International comparisons of childhood neoplasms. *Clin. Pediat.* (Phila.) 6:567-569, 1967.
9. Marigo, C., Muller, H., and Davies, J. N. P.: Survey of cancer in children admitted to a Brazilian charity hospital. *J. Nat. Cancer Inst.* 43:1231-1240, 1969.
10. Bras, G., Cole, H., Ashmeade-Dyar, A., and Watler, D. C.: Report on 151 childhood malignancies observed in Jamaica. *J. Nat. Cancer Inst.* 43:417-421, 1969.
11. Miller, R. W.: Persons with exceptionally high risk of leukemia. *Cancer Research* 27:2420-2423, 1967.
12. Miller, R. W.: Relation between cancer and congenital defects: an epidemiologic evaluation. *J. Nat. Cancer Inst.* 40:1079-1085, 1968.
13. Fraumeni, J. F., Jr. and Miller, R. W.: Epidemiology of human leukemia: recent observations. *J. Nat. Cancer Inst.* 38:593-605, 1967.
14. Fraumeni, J. F., Jr.: Constitutional disorders of man predisposing to leukemia and lymphoma. *Nat. Cancer Inst. Monogr.* 32:221-232, 1969.
15. Fraumeni, J. F., Jr.: Clinical epidemiology of leukemia. *Seminars in Hematology* 6:250-260, 1969.
16. Miller, R. W., Fraumeni, J. F., Jr. and Manning, M. D.: Association of Wilms' tumor with aniridia, hemihypertrophy and other congenital malformations. *New Eng. J. Med.* 270:922-927, 1964.
17. Fraumeni, J. F., Jr. and Miller, R. W.: Adrenocortical neoplasms with hemihypertrophy, brain tumors, and other disorders. *J. Pediat.* 70:129-138, 1967.
18. Fraumeni, J. F., Jr., Miller, R. W. and Hill, J. A.: Primary carcinoma of the liver in childhood: an epidemiologic study. *J. Nat. Cancer Inst.* 40:1087-1099, 1968.
19. Fraumeni, J. F., Jr., Geiser, C. F. and Manning, M. D.: Wilms' tumor and congenital hemihypertrophy: report of five new cases and review of literature. *Pediatrics* 40:886-899, 1967.
20. Fraumeni, J. F., Jr. and Glass, A. G.: Wilms' tumor and congenital aniridia. *JAMA* 206:825-828, 1968.

21. Miller, R. W.: Deaths from childhood leukemia and solid tumors among twins and other sibs in the United States, 1960-67. *J. Nat. Cancer Inst.* 46:203-209, 1971.
22. Snyder, A. L., Li, F. P., Henderson, E. S. and Todaro, G. J.: Possible inherited leukaemogenic factors in familial acute myelogenous leukaemia. *Lancet* 1:586-589, 1970.
23. Li, F. P. and Fraumeni, J. F., Jr.: Rhabdomyosarcoma in children: epidemiologic study and identification of a familial cancer syndrome. *J. Nat. Cancer Inst.* 43:1365-1373, 1969.
24. Li, F. P. and Fraumeni, J. F., Jr.: Soft-tissue sarcomas, breast cancer, and other neoplasms. A familial syndrome? *Ann. Intern. Med.* 71: 747-752, 1969.
25. Miller, R. W.: Transplacental chemical carcinogenesis in man. *J. Nat. Cancer Inst.* 47:-1169-1171, 1971.
26. Miller, R. W.: Etiology of childhood leukemia. Epidemiologic evidence. *Pediatric Clinics of North America* 13:267-277, 1966.
27. Herbst, A. L., Ulfelder, H. and Poskanzer, D. C.: Adenocarcinoma of the vagina: association of maternal stilbestrol therapy with tumor appearance in young women. *New Eng. J. Med.* 284:878-881, 1971.
28. Greenwald, P., Barlow, J. J., Nasca, D. C., et al: Vaginal cancer after maternal treatment with synthetic estrogen. *New Eng. J. Med.* 285: 390-392, 1971.

Viruses and Childhood Cancer

Joseph F. Fraumeni, Jr., M.D.

Since discoveries were made that viruses can cause leukemia and certain other cancers in laboratory animals, patterns of cancer in man have been examined in an effort to evaluate transmission by viruses.

Leukemia

In the 1960's the attention of cancer virologists and epidemiologists was drawn to childhood leukemia after "clusters" of this cancer were reported in certain communities and were considered to be evidence for a viral spread of disease. The most celebrated cluster was in Niles, Illinois, a suburb of Chicago.[1] In this community, eight cases of childhood leukemia occurred between 1957 and 1960, and all lived in the same residential neighborhood, corresponding to a Roman Catholic parish. Seven of the eight children were from Catholic families, and each either attended or had older siblings at the parochial grade school in the parish. There was no direct contact among the children or their families, but the rate of childhood leukemia in Niles during this period was about four to five times the usual frequency of this cancer. The eight cases also clustered within two separate, short intervals during the time period, and were associated with other unusual occurrences: a rheumatic-like disorder among many students in the parochial school, and an excess mortality from congenital heart disease in the community.[1]

What are the interpretations of such clusters? (a) They may represent foci of infection, or unusual exposure to unidentified environmental agents. (b) Some clusters may simply reflect the irregularity that occurs with relatively rare diseases, due to small numbers with a large standard deviation. (c) The gerrymandering of boundaries around cases in time and space may artificially produce certain clusters. (d) Exhaustive ascertainment of cases from one community may contrast with incomplete reporting from neighboring areas. (e) Clusters are influenced by demographic characteristics, particularly the recent in-migration of young people in suburban developments. (f) Finally, the

Joseph F. Fraumeni, Jr., M.D., *Head, Ecology Studies Section, Epidemiology Branch, National Cancer Institute, Bethesda, Maryland.*

play of chance results in some clusters, which inevitably occur over time in a certain proportion of communities in the United States.[2]

Therefore, the question should not be do clusters occur, but do they occur excessively. To evaluate this problem, statistical procedures were invented to examine the frequency of clustering within previously specified units of time and space. In general, there has been no excess of clustering over expectation in studies of various populations, whereas the same procedures detected enormous clustering for known infectious diseases such as polio and hepatitis.[2-5]

Another way to evaluate the viral hypothesis is to look at persons having unusual exposures. The risk of leukemia is not increased among spouses of leukemic patients, among persons *in utero* when the mother had leukemia, among children receiving neonatal exchange-transfusions, among persons exposed to leukemic animals, or in other situations that might reflect an infectious process.[2,6-9] The sibs of leukemic children have a four-fold excess of leukemia, but this increased risk may be due to genetic rather than environmental influences.[10]

In leukemia affecting mice, the viral transmission is not horizontal or contagious. It is vertical (from one generation to the next), in which the fetus is infected through the germ cells, placenta, or breast milk. The available evidence in human leukemia, however, does not support vertical transmission.[7-8] For example, there is no clear increase in leukemia among offspring of leukemic mothers, or in the mothers of children who develop leukemia at any age. When all reported occurrences of leukemia in parent and child were assembled from the literature, the frequency of leukemia in both mother and child was equal to the frequency in both father and child. Furthermore, the breast-feeding experiences of leukemic children are unremarkable. These findings suggest that leukemia viruses are not transmitted selectively from mother to child, either through the milk or placenta, as in the animal model.[7-8]

The contribution of viruses to leukemia may also be assessed by comparing its epidemiology with that for certain infectious diseases. Various workers have suggested, for example, that leukemia has similarities to the patterns for polio and for slow-virus infections. These models, however, do not hold up when critical epidemiologic features are compared with leukemia.[8]

These epidemiological observations, taken together, provide no convincing evidence for infectious transmission of leukemia in the usual sense.

Burkitt's Lymphoma

There is more evidence for a viral influence in Burkitt's lymphoma, which characteristically affects the jaw and rarely occurs outside of Central Africa.[11] On a safari through Africa, Burkitt found that this lymphoma had a restricted geographic distribution, dependent on the temperature and humidity of the area.

This observation suggested transmission of the disease by a mosquito-borne agent. The same geographic pattern occurs with malaria, which most workers now suspect is a contributing factor to the demographic features and origin of the lymphoma.[11] In addition, all patients with Burkitt's tumor have antibodies to a herpes-type virus (the Epstein-Barr or E-B virus), usually at high titer. The leading hypothesis now is that Burkitt's tumor results from combined infection with malaria and E-B virus.[12] In areas where lymphoma is common, malaria is holoendemic and 85% of the children have antibodies to E-B virus before age three. If interaction between the two infections causes lymphoma, it should occur at a very early age, when the malarial stress is greatest. Since Burkitt's lymphoma has a broad peak around seven years of age, there would be a variable latent period, averaging about five years. Unlike leukemia, Burkitt's lymphoma shows a tendency for time-space clustering of cases, which has suggested the possibility of an additional infectious agent with a short latent period.[12]

Hodgkin's Disease

In recent months, there has been much interest in a cluster of Hodgkin's disease among young adults in Albany, New York.[13] Unlike the leukemia cluster in Niles, the cases of Hodgkin's disease did not aggregate in time and space, but were discovered to have been previously associated with each other as high-school students. Some of the relationships were indirect, through contacts who did not develop the disease. The findings suggested person-to-person spread of an infectious agent, but could also be due to independent exposure of each patient to the same environmental factor. Also, the play of chance has not been entirely eliminated, since the relationships between cases may be what one would expect in linking any series of rare events. In any event, present knowledge of the epidemiology of Hodgkin's disease suggests that such clusters are very rare, and that heavy exposure to patients is not hazardous.

Breast Cancer from Breast Feeding

Carcinoma of the breast, the most common cancer of women, is now the subject of a controversy with implications to pediatric practice.[14] Virus particles have been detected recently in human milk and are felt by many workers to cause this cancer. These particles are structurally similar to the milk-transmitted virus which causes mammary cancer in mice; show reverse transcriptase activity which is characteristic of certain tumor viruses; and have been observed in a high proportion of milk samples from women whose near relatives had breast cancer. Since women with a positive family history are at increased risk of breast cancer, it has been suggested that such women, though healthy, should not breast feed their children because of the possible transmission of a cancer-causing virus.

This recommendation should be weighed against the evidence from man concerning possible viral spread from mother to daughter.[14] (a) In countries where breast feeding is common and prolonged, the rates for breast cancer are low. This finding is not due, as previously thought, to a protective influence of lactation on mother. (b) Familial aggregation of breast cancer occurs equally in the maternal and paternal lines. If the disease was maternally-transmitted, one would expect an excess of familial cases on the maternal side. (c) Mother-daughter occurrences of breast cancer are not associated with a history of breast feeding. (d) In the United States, breast feeding has declined in frequency, but the incidence of breast cancer has climbed. (e) Finally, the risk of this cancer is low among groups that favor breast feeding, such as rural dwellers, lower economic classes, and the foreign born. Thus, the available human data do not support the claim that breast cancer is related to breast feeding.[14]

Conclusions

The epidemiologic study of childhood cancer has succeeded in demonstrating relationships to a variety of characteristics, both inborn and acquired, but has failed to reveal an infectious mode of transmission. If viruses cause leukemia or other cancers among children in this country, they do so in a manner too subtle for epidemiologic detection.[7-8] Taking these observations into account, Huebner and Todaro of the National Cancer Institute proposed recently that all cells of the body contain latent viruses (called oncogenes) which are transmitted vertically and can cause cancer when activated by factors in the environment or host.[15] If true, cancer-causing viruses are not likely to be identified by the intensive investigation of clusters, but may be detected by laboratory studies on groups of children who carry an exceptional risk of cancer.[10,16,17]

References

1. Heath, C. W., Jr., and Manning, M. D.: Leukemia among children in a suburban community. *Amer. J. Med.* 34:796-812, 1963.
2. Fraumeni, J. F., Jr. and Miller, R. W.: Epidemiology of human leukemia: recent observations. *J. Nat. Cancer Inst.* 38:593-605, 1967.
3. Fraumeni, J. F., Jr., Ederer, F., and Handy, V. H.: Temporal-spatial distribution of childhood leukemia in New York State. *Cancer* 19:996-1000, 1966.
4. Glass, A. G., Hill, J. A., and Miller, R. W.: The significance of leukemia clusters. *J. Pediat.* 73:101-107, 1968.
5. Glass, A. G. and Mantel, N.: Lack of time-space clustering of childhood leukemia in Los Angeles County, 1960-1964. *Cancer Research* 29:1995-2001, 1969.
6. Miller, R. W.: Etiology of childhood leukemia. Epidemiologic evidence. *Pediatric Clinics of North America* 13:267-277, 1966.

7. Miller, R. W. and Fraumeni, J. F., Jr.: Leukemia houses. *Ann. Intern. Med.* 67:675-676, 1967.

8. Miller, R. W.: The viral etiology of leukemia: an epidemiologic evaluation, in *Proceedings of The International Conference on Leukemia-Lymphoma,* ed. C.J.D. Zarafonetis, Lea & Febiger, Philadelphia, 1968, pp. 23-29.

9. Fraumeni, J. F., Jr.: Clinical epidemiology of leukemia. Seminars in *Hematology* 6:250-260, 1969.

10. Miller, R. W.: Persons with exceptionally high risk of leukemia. *Cancer Research* 27:2420-2423, 1967.

11. Burkitt, D. P.: Etiology of Burkitt's lymphoma-an alternative hypothesis to a vectored virus. *J. Nat. Cancer Inst.* 42:19-28, 1969.

12. Morrow, R. H., Pike, M. C., Smith, P. G., Ziegler, J. L., and Kisuule, A.: Burkitt's lymphoma: a time-space cluster of cases in Bwamba County of Uganda. *Brit. Med. J.* 2:491-492, 1971.

13. Vianna, N. J., Greenwald, P., and Davies, J. N. P.: Extended epidemic of Hodgkin's disease in high-school students. *Lancet* 1:1209-1211, 1971.

14. Fraumeni, J. F., Jr. and Miller, R. W.: Breast cancer from breast-feeding. *Lancet* 2:1196-1197, 1971.

15. Huebner, R. J. and Todaro, G. J.: Oncogenes of RNA tumor viruses as determinants of cancer. *Proceedings of the National Academy of Sciences* 64:1087-1094, 1969.

16. Fraumeni, J. F., Jr.: Constitutional disorders of man predisposing to leukemia and lymphoma. *National Cancer Institute Monograph No. 32:*221-232, 1968.

17. Miller, R. W.: Relation between cancer and congenital defects: an epidemiologic evaluation. *J. Nat. Cancer Inst.* 40:1079-1085, 1968.

Immunological Aspects Observed in Childhood Malignancies; Rationale for Immunotherapy of These Tumors

Ronald B. Herberman, M.D.

Over the past few years there has been increasing evidence of tumor-associated antigens in a variety of human neoplasms, including childhood tumors. The major childhood tumors that have been studied and shown to give some evidence of tumor-associated antigens have included neuroblastoma, leukemia, sarcomas, and Burkitt's lymphoma. A variety of techniques have been used to make as much progress as we have to date. These techniques include: skin-testing for delayed hypersensitivity with extracts in the patients, various *in vitro* assays like colony inhibition and other forms of cytotoxicity reactions, lymphocyte stimulation, migration inhibition, and others. The two assays that we have spent most of our time working on in our laboratory, gathering evidence of this type, have been with the delayed hypersensitivity skin tests and with an *in vitro* cellular cytotoxicity reaction. The rationale for the skin-testing has been rather simple. If there are foreign antigens associated with the tumors and if there is a cell-mediated immune response to these antigens, one might expect to find delayed hypersensitivity reactions to the tumor cells or to extracts of the tumor cells, just as one gets a positive tuberculin reaction. We therefore proceeded to make membrane extracts of tumor cells, particularly from leukemia and lymphoma cells, and at the same time make comparable extracts of normal cells from the same patients. Most of the skin tests that we have performed have been in the autologous individuals, testing the extracts back into the same patients. But there has also been a fair amount of testing of extracts from one patient in other patients, looking for common antigens within a particular disease.

Figure 1 is a photograph of positive delayed reactions to tumor extracts. The delayed hypersensitivity reactions do not photograph very well. The main thing that we have been looking for has been the appearance of erythema and induration, usually reaching a maximum between 30-48 hours after inoculation

Ronald B. Herberman, M.D., *Head, Cellular and Tumor Immunology Section, Laboratory of Cell Biology, National Cancer Institute, Bethesda, Maryland.*

15

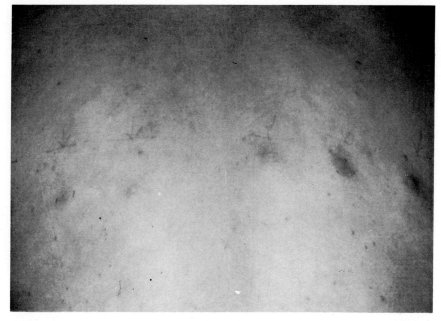

Figure 1.

of the material. With most of the skin tests that we did during the first year of the study, punch biopsies were taken to confirm that these reactions were similar in histology to that of a tuberculin reaction and to other forms of classical delayed hypersensitivity reactions.

The histological hallmark of delayed hypersensitivity reactions has been the appearance of mononuclear cells, mainly clustered around small vessels in the epidermis (Fig. 2). This type of reaction is really indistinguishable from what one sees with a classical delayed hypersensitivity reaction.

One of the diseases which we looked at rather extensively at first was Burkitt's lymphoma. Burkitt's tumor is about the most common form of childhood malignancy in certain regions of Africa. There have been many suggestions over the past several years that there may be a viral etiology for this disease and also perhaps some type of host defense mechanism against the disease, particularly with the occurrence of spontaneous regressions of the tumor.

When skin tests were performed on patients soon after the original biopsy, when the tumor was still present and before chemotherapy, only 1 of over 30 patients gave positive delayed hypersensitivity reactions to tumor extract. This did not appear to be due to general unreactivity in that simultaneous skin tests with tuberculin and other skin test antigens were positive in the same patients.

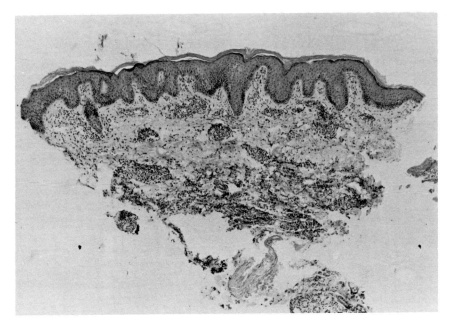

Figure 2.

After the patients were treated with cyclophosphamide or other forms of chemotherapy and went into remission, the skin tests were repeated or performed for the first time; the results were quite different. At this time, there were many positive skin tests to extracts made from the tumor cells but not to the leucocytes of the same patients. If one analyzes the incidence of positive reactions in patients according to the rate of relapse, there was no apparent association (Fig. 3). The patients that were skin-test-positive in remission relapsed at a rate of 44%; the patients who were skin-test-negative relapsed at a rate of 50%, which is not a significant difference. Similarly, when we analyzed for mortality, about 20% of the patients died in each of these groups. The most striking correlation, which has continued to persist as the numbers get larger, is that the patients in remission who give a positive skin test tend to remain in remission significantly longer than those who give a negative skin test. The presence of positive reactivity seems to have some prognostic implications. Seven of the patients who were skin-test-positive in remission relapsed, and in all of these, around the time of relapse, the skin test changed from positive to negative.

We have performed similar assays on patients in the United States with acute lymphocytic leukemia and acute myelogenous leukemia.

Again, patients were tested with extracts either from the leukemic cells or, for control purposes, from the remission cells of the same patients (Fig.4). In

SKIN TEST WITH BURKITT'S TUMOR
CORRELATION WITH CLINICAL STATUS

	Skin Test	
	Positive	Negative
Relapse rate	11/25 (44%)	9/18 (50%)
Mortality	5/25 (20%)	4/18 (22%)
Remission Duration (mean in weeks)	25	16

Figure 3.

patients who were known to be nonanergic, i.e., those who had delayed hypersensitivity reactions to some recall antigens, there was a correlation of skin reactivity to tumor extracts with the clinical state. During the leukemic phase of the disease, when tumor cells were present, only about one-third of the patients gave positive skin test reactions. In tests performed in remission, most of the patients had positive skin reactions to tumor extracts. This has been the case both with patients who have acute lymphocytic leukemia and patients with acute myelogenous leukemia. All of the tests that we have done so far with remission extracts have been negative. We have followed several patients serially,

SKIN TESTS - ACUTE LYMPHOCYTIC LEUKEMIA

(Nonanergic Patients)

Test Material	Skin Test Results	Tests Performed in	
		Leukemic Phase	Remission
Autologous Leukemia Cell Membranes	Positive	5	5
	Negative	9	1
Autologous Remission Cell Membranes	Positive	NT*	0
	Negative	NT	6

*NT = not tested

Figure 4.

repeating the same tests as the patients went from remission to relapse and back to remission; in these patients there was almost a complete correspondance of skin reactivity to the tumor extract with the state of the disease. In several of the patients, the skin test converted several weeks before the clinical conversion was obvious.

There have been several *in vitro* assays that have been successfully used to study tumor immunity, including lymphocyte stimulation and various types of cytotoxicity reactions. The Hellstroms in Seattle, for instance, have done extensive studies on neuroblastoma and some other diseases using the colony inhibition technique. The major assay which we focused upon *in vitro* was a cellular cytotoxicity test. Figure 5 indicates how cells were prepared for use in this assay.

Heparinized peripheral blood was obtained from the patients and passed through a nylon column to separate out the lymphocytes; or the lymphocytes have been separated on a Ficoll-Hypaque density gradient. The red cells were removed by settling with Plasmagel and the lymphocytes were then harvested. This provided the attacking lymphocyte population. This type of separation often pertained also to the target cells taken from the peripheral blood of the

PREPARATION OF CELLS FOR DETECTION OF
CELL MEDIATED IMMUNITY *In Vitro*

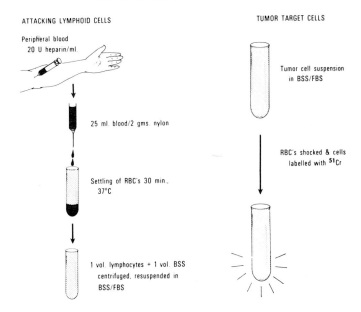

ATTACKING LYMPHOID CELLS

TUMOR TARGET CELLS

Peripheral blood
20 U heparin/ml.

Tumor cell suspension
in BSS/FBS

25 ml. blood/2 gms. nylon

RBC's shocked & cells
labelled with ^{51}Cr

Settling of RBC's 30 min.,
37°C

1 vol. lymphocytes + 1 vol. BSS
centrifuged, resuspended in
BSS/FBS

Figure 5.

leukemia patients. The target cells were labelled with chromium-51 to use as a measure of cytotoxicity.

The assay consisted of mixing the attacking lymphoid cells from the patients or from control individuals with the chromium-51 labelled tumor cells, at a ratio of 60:1. There were control dishes in which no attacking lymphocytes were added or in which control lymphocytes were added. The mixtures were incubated together at 37 degrees for 4 hours and the supernatants from these cultures were then assayed for the amount of chromium released into the supernatant. This is a very accurate indicator of the amount of killing of the cells which goes on during this period of time.

Table 1 is a summary of some of the reactions that we have seen in patients with acute lymphocytic leukemia and patients with acute myelogenous leukemia. We have found positive reactions in both diseases. This reactivity appears to be specific, in that one can get positive reactions to the frozen tumor cells but not to remission lymphocytes or granulocytes taken from the same patients. If one tries to correlate reactivity with the clinical state of the patient at the time the test is done, one sees a rather different picture than was seen with the skin tests. With both ALL and AML, the reactivity was just as great, if not greater, in patients who were in relapse than in patients who were in remission. The numbers are still not large enough to make this a significant difference.

One of the things which we have tried to do with this test, in addition to looking for autologous reactivity of the patients themselves, is to screen populations – family members and unrelated control individuals – for possible reactivity against antigens that might be associated with the tumor. This is particularly important in terms of investigating the possible viral etiology for leukemia. If there is a common virus which is present in the environment to which many people are exposed, one then might predict that family members or even unrelated normal individuals would have immunological reactivity to antigens on the leukemia cells. There is ample precedent for this type of reactivity in animal systems, particularly in the mouse. To control this situation

TABLE 1. Lymphocyte Cytotoxicity Reactions of Patients with Leukemia Against Autochthonous Blast Cells

Patients	Reactivity to Autologous Blasts (Tests positive*/Total number of Tests)
ALL, relapse	2/3
ALL, remission	3/9
AML, relapse	2/3
AML, remission	2/10

*% lysis significantly different from background release, $p < 0.05$.

as much as we possibly could, we focused upon studies in patients with acute leukemia, who had identical twins available. We could then simultaneously look at reactivity of the individuals themselves, their identical twin, and other family members against two types of target cells; the leukemic cells and the control cells from the normal twin.

Figure 6 illustrates a representative study of this type. The patient had acute lymphocytic leukemia and, at the time of the study, there were malignant cells in lymph nodes but not in his spleen, nor in his peripheral blood. Therefore, from the patient himself, we had tumor cells plus two sources of control cells. In addition, we had the lymphocytes from the normal twin. It was found that the patient's normal lymphocytes had cytotoxic reactivity, that was significantly higher than the controls, against his tumor cells, but not against his normal spleen cells, nor against his remission lymphocytes, nor against the lymphocytes of his normal twin. The normal twin also had the same pattern of reactivity: positive reactions with the tumor cells but not with the other cell types. With further studies along this line, we have found that not only the identical twins themselves but also family members – mother, father, siblings – and a number of unrelated individuals have reactivity against the cells from the leukemic twin but not for the comparable cells from the normal identical twin, suggesting that there is sensitization in the environment against the antigens associated with leukemia. One of the intriguing observations from this has been that in some studies the reactivity has not only been against the leukemia cells of the patients but also against the remission leukocytes from the patients with leukemia. In

LYMPHOCYTE CYTOTOXICITY IN IDENTICAL TWINS

PATIENT: A.M., lymphocytic lymphoma with leukemia

^{51}Cr-Target Cells	% Cytotoxicity ($\pm$ S.E.M.)	
	Patient's Lymphocytes	Normal Twin's Lymphocytes
Lymphoma	4.1 (0.68)**	5.18 (2.24)*
Spleen cells, patient	-1.2 (0.8)	-1.0 (0.54)
Lymphocytes, patient	0.99 (0.42)	0.96 (0.57)
Lymphocytes, normal twin	-0.24 (0.43)	-0.05 (0.4)

   * Significant, at 0.05 level

  ** Significant, p <0.05

Figure 6.

those studies, the cells from the leukemic twin were morphologically indistinguishable from those of the normal twin, yet there was a qualitative difference in the reactivity that was seen, with positive cytotoxicity against the remission cells from the leukemic, and no reactivity against the normal twin. This suggested that some of the antigens associated with the leukemic process may even be present when the patient is in clinical remission. Sensitization of patients and other individuals to a virus associated with leukemia would be a leading hypothesis to explain the type of reactivity that we have seen.

In terms of the usefulness of these tests in a more general sense, the fact that assays like this and the others that I have mentioned can show the presence of both tumor-associated antigens in these diseases and also immune reactivity of the patients against these tumors provides a strong basis — or a rationale, at least — for immunotherapeutic manipulations in patients with cancer. If there is an antigen against which one can direct an immunotherapeutic approach, if there is a potential at least of the patient's responding immunologically against the tumor, then there is a very good rationale for trying immunotherapy. One of the major problems with immunotherapy is that up until now it has been largely empirical. If someone decides upon a particular type of manipulation, they proceed to try it out on some patients. Most of these studies have not been accompanied by any measurement of immune activity that may be produced in the patients. Furthermore, these studies have not usually been well-controlled. Assays of immunological reactivity to tumor antigens should provide important help in monitoring any attempts at immunotherapy, either in animals or in man. During an immunotherapy trial, one can also ask the question: "Are there changes being produced in these assays by the immunological manipulation?" If one cannot detect any change in the immunological assays, there may be little hope that one will be able to succeed in the therapeutic scheme. There is a study going on now at the National Cancer Institute of injecting patients with acute lymphocytic leukemia with allogeneic leukemia cells and/or BCG. The patients are being monitored with three assays for immune reactivity. There has been some indication that stimulation does occur by these modalities. The work is still quite preliminary, but it is promising; and this type of testing should give us a lot of insight into what is going on.

The other point that I would like to bring out, which is illustrated by the different types of clinical correlations which we have seen with the skin tests and the cellular cytotoxicity, is that if one performs two or more different immunological assays simultaneously on the same patient, one can often see different results in the different assays. We have studied a series of acute leukemia patients with these two assays and with lymphocyte stimulation; there has been a very poor correlation among the three assays, with only the skin test correlating with the clinical state of the patient. At the present state of our knowledge, selection of only one assay to follow the immunological responsiveness of the patient probably will not be sufficient. Until we get a better understanding of the interrelationships between each of these assays and the relationship of each assay to the *in vivo* situation, there will be a need for this type of comparative testing.

References

1. Fass, L., Herberman, R. B., and Ziegler, J.: Delayed cutaneous hypersensitivity reactions to autologous extracts of Burkitt's lymphoma cells. *New Eng. J. Med.* 282 :776, 1970.
2. Oren, M. and Herberman, R.: Delayed cutaneous hypersensitivity reactions to membrane extracts of human tumour cells. *Clin. Exp. Immunol.* 9:45, 1971.
3. Bluming, A. Z., Ziegler, J. L., Fass, L., and Herberman, R. B.: Delayed cutaneous sensitivity reactions to autologous Burkitt lymphoma protein extracts: results of a prospective two and a half year study. *Clin. Exp. Immunol.* (in press), 1971.
4. Herberman, R. B., and Rosenberg, E. B.: *Cellular cytotoxicity reactions to human leukemia associated antigens.* Proceedings of the Fifth International Symposium on Comparative Leukemia Research, (in press), 1972.
5. Rosenberg, E. B., Herberman, R. B., Levine, P. H., Halterman, R., McCoy, J. L., and Wunderlich, J. R.: Lymphocyte cytotoxicity reactions to leukemia associated antigens in identical twins. *Int. J. Cancer,* (in press), 1972.
6. Leventhal, B. G., Halterman, R. H., Rosenberg, E. B., and Herberman, R. B.: Immune reactivity of leukemia patients to autologous blast cells. *Cancer Research,* (in press), 1972.

Clinical Manifestations and Differential Diagnosis of Malignant Solid Tumors of Childhood

Kjell Koch, M.D., M.S. (Peds)

General Considerations

Before referring more specifically to the clinical manifestations of malignant tumors of childhood, it is important to reemphasize the fact that there are differences between the adult and pediatric population in relation to type of lesions, incidence, as well as clinical behavior. It has already been pointed out that the malignant tumors commonly seen in adult life, such as carcinoma of the gastrointestinal tract, lung, breast and female genital tract, are either absent or are seldom seen below the age of sixteen years.[1-3] Similarly, the embryonal tumors characteristic of the pediatric age group are exceedingly rare in adults. Within the pediatric age group there are changes in the incidence of the various types of malignant disorders according to different age periods.[4] During infancy and up to approximately eight years the predominant malignancies are leukemia, neuroblastoma, Wilm's tumor, retinoblastoma and sarcomas of the soft tissue. Neoplasms of the central nervous system are more prevalent between five and ten years of age, and after puberty Hodgkin's disease, osteogenic sarcoma and Ewing's tumor may be seen more frequently than in earlier years. According to sites, tumors in childhood are more commonly found in the hematopoietic tissues, retroperitoneal area, intracranial cavity, eye and orbit, skin and soft tissues, and in the bones.[1]

The early diagnosis is unfortunately difficult to achieve in most of the childhood neoplasms because usually the disease is rather silent or insidious in onset and often, when overt symptoms and signs have appeared, the process by then may be quite advanced and difficult to control. As compared to adults, systemic manifestations of cancer are less frequent in the initial states and, at times, even in the presence of a large tumoral mass, there may be no significant

Kjell Koch, M.D., M.S. (Peds) *Department of Pediatrics, University of Miami School of Medicine, Miami, Florida.* *

*This work was supported in part by the Florida Regional Medical Program, Grant No. 33.

anemia or loss of weight. Nevertheless, a stationary growth curve may represent an important initial sign of a malignant process. An example of this situation is neuroblastoma.

In general and from a clinical point of view, childhood solid malignancies, with the exclusion of intracranial and intrathoracic lesions, manifest by the presence of an abnormal mass or organomegaly which may attain a large size in a relatively short period of time. The abnormal mass may be more evident in regions such as the neck, abdomen and extremities where inspection and palpation are the primary tools of detection. Intracranial and intrathoracic neoplasms usually manifest by symptoms and signs resulting from the compression and destruction of the regional tissues, but actual visualization of the abnormal mass may only be possible through radiological scanning, or exploratory surgical procedures. Not uncommonly, the first manifestations of the malignant disease are related to the appearance of the metastases, and the site of the primary lesion at times may be difficult or impossible to establish.

It is not intended in this presentation to discuss the laboratory aspects of the various malignant tumors of childhood. Nevertheless, it is pertinent to stress in general terms the importance of the hematological evaluation. Anemia, thrombocytopenia or changes in the white blood elements may be a cardinal part of the clinical picture. Certainly a bone marrow examination is helpful, not only because it may give the exact diagnosis as in cases of neuroblastoma and obviously in leukemia, but it may serve also to define the degree of tumoral involvement. The study of the urine may reveal hematuria in patients with tumors of the kidney or lower genitourinary tract, and abnormal levels of urinary catecholamines are usually found in patients with neuroblastoma.[5] Radiological and nuclear medicine procedures are certainly most important in the diagnostic work-up, and these aspects will be discussed in other sections of this symposium. It is important to stress the concept that regardless of the clinical and laboratory data which may be highly indicative of a specific disorder, a definite diagnosis cannot be made until adequate histopathological studies are completed.

Topographic Distribution

Table 1 represents the regional distribution of 159 cases of malignant neoplasm including leukemia, seen in the Department of Pediatrics, University of Miami, between 1962 and 1971. Of this material 75 were leukemia and 84 were solid tumors. Of this, the majority occurred in the abdomen (32 cases). The second next common location was the head (23 cases). The rest of the tumors were distributed almost equally between the neck, chest, pelvic area and extremities. The two most common specific solid malignant neoplasms were Wilm's tumor and neuroblastoma.

TABLE 1. Topographic Distribution of Malignant Tumors of Childhood
(159 Cases)
University of Miami (1962-71)

Type	No. of Cases	H	N	C	A	P	E	S
LEUKEMIA	75							75
SOLID TUMORS	84	23	7	8	32	5	7	2
Wilm's	16	–	–	–	16	–	–	–
Neuroblastoma	11	–	–	1	10	–	–	–
CNS tumors	10	10	–	–	–	–	–	–
Hodgkin's D.	10	–	6	3	–	–	1	–
Lymphosarcoma	9	1	1	3	2	–	2	–
Rhabdomyosarcoma	9	2	–	1	–	4	2	–
Histiocytosis	8	5	–	–	1	–	–	–
Retinoblastoma	5	5	–	–	–	–	–	–
Hepatoma	1	–	–	–	1	–	–	–
Sarcoma, undif.	1	–	–	–	–	–	1	–
Teratoma, malig.	1	–	–	–	–	1	–	–
Renal cell Ca	1	–	–	–	1	–	–	–
Adrenal cell Ca	1	–	–	–	1	–	–	–
Ewing's sarcoma	1	–	–	–	–	–	1	–
Total	159	23	7	8	32	5	7	77

H=head; N=neck; C=chest; A=abdomen; P=pelvic; E=extremities; S=systemic.

Malignant Tumors of the Head

The most common malignant tumors of the head are the intracranial neoplasms.[6] (See Table 2) This subject is discussed in detail by Dr. Brown in another section.

Primary malignant lesions of the skull are rare, the most important being osteogenic sarcoma and reticuloendotheliosis. Metastatic lesions in this location may derive from neuroblastoma and more rarely from Wilm's tumor. Usually, these skull lesions may be initially silent unless they extend to the external or internal soft tissue regions. In the head, extracranial malignant tumors are rather rare; nevertheless, tumors of this region are more frequently seen in the ocular or orbital areas. A cat's eye pupillary reflex should alert one to the possibility of a retinoblastoma,[7] which represents the most common intraocular tumor. The orbit is one of the most common sites for rhabdomyosarcoma,[8] and clinical manifestations of this tumor may be in the form of swelling and proptosis. The presence of subconjunctival hemorrhage is highly suggestive of metastatic neuroblastoma. An orbital lesion may also represent reticuloendotheliosis,[9] especially if proptosis is associated with bone lesions and diabetes insipidus

TABLE 2. Malignant Tumors of the Head in Childhood
University of Miami (1962-71)

Site	Type	No. Cases	Clinical Features
INTRACRANIAL	CNS tumors	10	Increased intracranial P.
SKULL	Osteogenic S.	0	Initially silent unless
	Histiocytosis	3	extension to adjacent
	Metastatic	–	soft tissues
EXTRACRANIAL			
Eye, orbit	Retinoblastoma	5	Cat's eye sign
	Rhabdomyosarcoma	1	Proptosis
	Neuroblastoma, metast.	–	Hemorrhage
	Histiocytosis		
Nasopharynx	Rhabdomyosarcoma	1	Nasal obstruction
Parasinuses	Carcinoma	0	Epistaxis, muco-sanguinolent
	Reticulum cell S.	1	discharge
Salivary G.	Mixed tumor	0	Mass; pain; facial palsy
	Muco epidermoid Ca	0	
Oral region	Rhabdomyosarcoma	0	Mass; macroglosia; "floating
	Lymphoma (Burkitt's)	0	teeth"
	Histiocytosis	2	
Tonsil	Lymphosarcoma	0	Mass
Soft parts	Rhabdomyosarcoma	0	Nodule
	Metastatic neuroblast	–	
	Total	23	

(Hand-Schuller-Christian syndrome). A Horner's syndrome certainly should suggest the possibility of a posterior mediastinal mass.

Nasal obstruction, especially associated with epistaxis or muco-sanguinolent discharge may indicate the presence of a malignant lesion involving the naso-pharynx or the para-sinuses. The most important malignant tumor involving this region is rhabdomyosarcoma, although other types such as carcinoma and reticulum cell sarcoma may also occur.[1-10] The differential diagnosis should include sinusitis and benign neoplasias such as nasal polyps, papillomas and juvenile angiofibroma. The latter is seen usually in teen-age males.[11]

Malignancies of the salivary glands are rare; the cardinal clinical manifestations of a mixed tumor of the parotid are enlargement of the gland, pain, and facial paralysis. Chronic parotiditis should be considered in the differential diagnosis.[12]

Very few malignant tumors arise in the oral cavity, but the most representative are rhabdomyosarcoma,[1] Burkitt's lymphoma[13] and reticulo-endotheliosis.[9] Manifestations of these disorders may be in the form of a mass or swelling, macroglosia and "floating" teeth. Tonsils are rarely the site of a primary malignant neoplasm, although lymphoma may occur in this region.

Malignant Tumors of the Neck

In the neck most of the abnormal masses are non-tumoral, being represented usually by adenitis of infectious origin. (See Table 3) Tuberculosis, cat's scratch fever, and infectious mononucleosis should be considered in the differential diagnosis. It is pertinent to point out that a mass in the neck may be due to a thyroglossal cyst, brachial cleft cyst, teratoma, thymic cyst and hygroma colli. Among the malignant neoplasms involving the lymph nodes of the cervical region, the lymphoma group is the most important one. The possibilities of neuroblastoma, rhabdomyosarcoma, and reticuloendotheliosis should also be considered as well as cancer of the thyroid.[14]

Malignant Tumors of the Chest

In the chest most of the primary malignant neoplasms arise from the mediastinum. (See Table 4) Extrathoracic malignant tumors are rather rare, although several types may arise from the soft tissues, breast, ribs, spine and axillary nodes. Primary tumors of the lungs are rare,[15] this organ being more commonly the site of metastatic lesions derived from several neoplasms such as Wilm's tumor, osteogenic sarcoma, Ewing's sarcoma, amelanotic melanoma, rhabdomyosarcoma, lymphoma and neuroblastoma.[1]

The mediastinal tumors may occupy the anterior, middle or posterior mediastinum.[16] If the location of the abnormal mass is anterior, the differential diagnosis involves thymic enlargement, which is usually secondary to hyperplasia or congenital thymic cyst. Thymoma is extremely rare in the pediatric population. The second most common lesion of the anterior mediastinum is teratoma. This tumor frequently exhibits calcification which helps in differentiating from thymus and also may produce tracheal compression. Lymphoma, although usually more frequent in the middle mediastinum, may also involve the anterior region. Rarely a mass here is due to lymphangioma, pericardial cyst, intrathoracic goiter or diaphragmatic hernia.

TABLE 3. Malignant Tumors of the Neck in Childhood
University of Miami (1962-71)

Site	Type	No. Cases	Clinical Features
Lymph node	Lymphoma	6	Cervical Mass
	Rhapdomyosarcoma	0	
	Histiocytosis	0	
	Neuroblastoma	0	
	Metastatic	–	
Thyroid	Carcinoma	0	Nodule
Spine	Reticulum cell S.	1	Neurological

TABLE 4. Malignant Tumors of the Chest in Childhood
University of Miami (1962-71)

Site	Type	No. Cases	Clinical Features
EXTRATHORACIC			
Soft tissue	Sarcoma	0	Mass
Breast	Rhabdomyosarcoma	1	
	Carcinoma	0	
Rib	Chondrosarcoma	0	
	Ewing's Sarcoma	0	Pain, local heat, erythema
Lymph node	Hodgkin's	1	Mass
INTRATHORACIC			
Lung, pleura	Metastatic	–	Respiratory syndrome;
	Carcinoma	0	pain
	Sarcoma	0	
Mediastinum			
ant.	Teratoma	0	
	Thymoma	0	
med.	Lymphoma	5	Sup. mediastinal S.;
pos.	Neuroblastoma	1	Horner's Syndrome
Heart	Rhabdomyosarcoma	0	Pain; dyspnea; cardiac
	Lymphoma	0	failure; sup. & inf. vena cava obst.
	Total	8	

The most frequent malignant neoplasm in the middle mediastinum is lymphoma, especially lymphosarcoma. Hodgkin's disease is usually less common, although its incidence begins to increase after ten years of age. Differential diagnosis should include inflammatory conditions of the lymph nodes such as tuberculosis and viral adenitis. Sarcoidosis may occur but is rare in the pediatric age group. Aneuryms of the pulmonary arteries and congenital anomalies of the great vessels may also be responsible for masses in this region and should be considered in the differential diagnosis.

In the *posterior mediastinum,* the most frequent neoplasms are neurogenic tumors, such as neuroblastoma and ganglioneuroma. Differential diagnosis should also include gastorenteric cysts, neurenteric cysts, bronchogenic cysts, and lesions of the esophagus, such as achalasia, and cardiospasm.

Clinically, the clue manifestations of mediastinal tumors may be those of a superior mediastinal syndrome or a Horner's syndrome. Although many of the mentioned lesions may have characteristic radiological features, an exact diagnosis is made only through biopsy, which is best obtained by exploratory thoracotomy. We have found that mediastinoscopy in many cases is unsatisfactory in providing adequate specimen.

The heart is seldom a site of a primary malignant tumor, although rhabdomyosarcomas and malignant teratomas have been reported to occur in this organ.[17-18]

Malignant Tumors of the Abdomen

In the abdomen, we find the most characteristic malignant tumors of the pediatric age group.[18a] (See Table 5) It is pertinent to remember that most abdominal masses are retroperitoneal (70%) as compared to intra-abdominal masses (30%). The organs most frequently responsible for intra-abdominal masses are the liver and the spleen. Most of the hepatic enlargements are related to inflammatory conditions. Primary malignant tumors of the liver are rare, hepatoma[19] being the most important one. Metastatic lesions involving this organ are certainly more frequent than primary neoplasms and they may derive from a variety of tumors, such as Wilm's, neuroblastoma and lymphoma. The spleen is seldom the site of a primary malignancy in childhood, but lymphoma has been reported, and should be considered in the differential diagnosis of splenomegalies.

Tumors of the gastrointestinal tract are uncommon in children, as compared to adults. Actually, the most common tumor of the alimentary tract in childhood is the juvenile polyp.[20] a benign lesion. Among the malignant tumors lymphosarcoma is the most important one and may occur especially involving

TABLE 5. Malignant Tumors of the Abdomen in Childhood
University of Miami (1962-71)

Site	Type	No. Cases	Clinical Features
INTRAABDOMINAL			
Liver	Hepatoma	1	Hepatomegaly
Metastatic	Metastatic	–	
Spleen	Lymphoma	0	Splenomegaly
GI Tract	Lymphoma	0	Mass; pain;
	Carcinoma	0	hemorrhage; obstruction
	Histiocytosis	1	
	Carcinoid*	0	*Carcinoid syndrome
RETROPERITONEAL			
Renal	Wilm's tumor	16	Mass, hypertension;
	Hypernehroma	1	hematuria
	Lymphoma	1	
Adrenal &	Neuroblastoma	10	Mass; pain; weight loss;
sympathetic	Adrenal cell Ca	1	functional manifestations
Lymph node	Lymphoma	1	Mass
Paravertebral	Teratoma	0	Mass
	Total	32	

the small intestine, producing obstructive manifestations. Cancer of the colon is very rare and may be related to polyposis or ulcerative colitis.[22]

Most of the abdominal masses occur in the retroperitoneum and the kidney represents the most common site. It is pertinent to point out that the most frequent causes of renal enlargement are: first, hydronephrosis; second, Wilm's tumor; and third, cystic disease. Hypernephroma is exceedingly rare under 30 years of age.[23] Other malignant tumors involving the retroperitoneal area include neuroblastoma, lymphoma and teratoma.

Clinically there are no pathognomonic signs for the various malignancies which one may encounter in the abdomen. Nevertheless, the association of an abdominal mass with hypertension or hematuria is highly suspicious of Wilm's tumor.[24] These changes are less common in neuroblastoma.[25] The physical characteristics of the palpable mass may be at times helpful. Usually the Wilm's tumor has a smooth spherical appearance and rarely crosses the midline; whereas the neuroblastoma may have an irregular nodular outline and not uncommonly crosses the midline.

Malignant Tumors of the Pelvic Region

In the pelvic region primary malignancies are rather rare in the pediatric population. (See Table 6) Rhabdomyosarcoma[26] represents the most important tumor and may arise from the bladder, prostate or vagina. Clinically, obstructive signs of the genitourinary tract as well as hematuria, may be one of the first

TABLE 6. Malignant Tumors of the Pelvic Area in Childhood University of Miami (1962-71)

Site	Type	No. Cases	Clinical Features
Bladder	Rhabdomyosarcoma	3	Hematuria; obstruction; pain; infection; mass
Male organs			
Testis	Embryonal Ca	0	Enlargement; hard
	Teratoma	0	mass
	Lymphosarcoma	0	
Prostate	Rhabdomyosarcoma	1	
Female organs			
Ovary	Adenocarcinoma	0	Pain; mass
	Teratoma	1	
	Dysgerminoma	0	
Uterus	Carcinoma	0	Hemorrhage
Vagina, vulva	Sarcoma Botryoides	0	Polypoid mass
	Melanoma	0	
Sacrococygeal	Teratoma	0	Mass
	Total	5	

manifestations before evidence of a pelvic mass can be demonstrated. We have seen one case of Rhabdomyosarcoma occuring in a boy in whom the initial problem was that of an apparently severe urinary infection secondary to lower urinary obstruction. In general primary malignancies of the female and male reproductive organs are rare in the pediatric age group. Clinically, an ovarian tumor may manifest by vomiting, abdominal pain and the presence of low abdominal or pelvic mass.[26a]

Malignant Tumors of the Extremities

In the area of the extremities, primary malignant tumors may derive from the skin and subcutaneous tissues, lymph nodes, muscles, and bone. (See Table 7) We have seen several patients with lymphomas, including lymphosarcoma and Hodgkin's disease, with primary involvement of the femoral lymph nodes. In the muscle, rhabdomyosarcoma is the most important malignant tumor. The initial presentation is that of an abnormal swelling or mass, or a rather diffuse indurated lesion which may suggest vasculitis, lymphedema or cellulitis. Abnormal swelling, pain, local heat and erythema, which may simulate osteomyelitis, may be the initial manifestations of bone neoplasms such as osteogenic sarcoma or Ewing's tumor.

Although more common in later life, primary reticulum cell sarcoma of the bone may occur also in the pediatric age group with a regional distribution similar to Ewing's tumor. A variety of other osseous lesions must be considered in the differential diagnosis of a primary bone neoplasm. Some of these lesions may be related to metastatic neuroblastoma, leukemia, reticuloendotheliosis,

TABLE 7. Malignant Tumors of the Extremities in Childhood
University of Miami (1962-71)

Site	Type	No. Cases	Clinical Features
Skin, subcut.	Melanoma	0	Dark, nodular lesion
	Carcinoma	0	Mass
	Fibrosarcoma	0	
	Rhabdomyosarcoma	0	
	Liposarcoma	0	
	Sarcoma, undif.	1	
Lymph node	Lymphoma	3	Mass
	Metastatic	–	
Muscle	Rhabdomyosarcoma	2	Mass
Bone	Osteogenic S.	0	Mass; local heart; erythema
	Ewing's sarcoma	1	pain
	Reticulum cell S.	0	
	Metastatic	–	
	Total	7	

benign bone tumors, injuries, infections or systemic non-neoplestic disorders.[28-30]

Summary

Early diagnosis of cancer in childhood requires knowledge of the initial clinical manifestations of a variety of malignant neoplasms. The incidence of the various types of malignancies changes according to different age groups. During infancy and up to approximately eight years of age the most predominant forms of cancer are leukemia, neuroblastoma, Wilm's tumor, retinoblastoma and sarcomas of the soft tissues; central nervous system neoplasms are more commonly seen in the five to ten years group. Hodgkin's disease, osteogenic sarcoma and Ewing's tumor are more likely to occur after puberty. Excluding brain tumors, which are usually related to signs of increased intracranial pressure, the majority of the malignant solid tumors become apparent by the presence of an abnormal mass which may attain large size in a relatively short period of time. Intrathoracic masses may be suspected in the presence of respiratory, cardiovascular symptomatology or a Horner's syndrome. A regional approach may be helpful in the differential diagnosis of malignant tumors of childhood.

References

1. Dargeon, H. W.: Tumors of Childhood, New York:Paul B. Hoeber, Inc., 1960.
2. Andersen, D. H.: Tumors of infancy and childhood. I. A survey of those in the Pathology Laboratory of the Babies Hospital during the years 1935-1950. *Cancer* 4:890, 1951.
3. Peller, S.: Cancer in Childhood and Youth, Bristol: John Wright & Sons, 1960.
4. Ariel, I. M., and Park, G. T.: *Cancer and Applied Diseases of Infancy and Childhood* Boston:Little, Brown and Co., 1960.
5. Gitlow, S. E. *et al.*: Diagnosis of Neuroblastoma by qualitative and quantitative determination of catecholamine metabolites in the urine. *Cancer* 25:1377, June, 1970.
6. Bailey, P., Buchanan, D. N., and Bucy, P. C.: *Intracranial Tumors of Infancy and Childhood* Chicago: University of Chicago Press, 1939.
7. Reese, A. B.: *Tumors of the Eye*, 2nd Ed., New York:Paul B. Hoeber, Inc., 1963.
8. Stobbe, G. D. and Dargeon, H. W.: Embryonal rhabdomyosarcoma of the head and neck in children and adolescents, *Cancer* 3:826, 1950.
9. Dargeon, W. K.: Reticuloendotheliosis in Childhood. A clinical survey. Springfield, Ill.:Charles C Thomas, 1966.
10. Ringertz, N.: Pathology of malignant tumors arising in the nasal, and para-nasal cavities and maxilla. *Acta oto-laryng,* Suppl. 27, 1938.
11. Pimpinella, R. J.: The nasopharyngeal angiofibroma in the adolescent male. *J. Pediat.* 64:260, 1964.
12. Kauffman, S. L. and Sout, A. P.: Tumors of the major salivary glands in children. *Cancer* 16:1317, 1963.
13. Burkitt, D. P. and Kyalwazi, S. K.: African (Burkitt's) Lymphoma: Characteristic features of Response to Therapy. *Neoplasia in Childhood* Year Book Med. Publishers, Inc., 1969.

14. Winship, T. and Rosvoll, R. V.: Childhood thyroid carcinoma. *Cancer* 14:734, 1961.
15. Cayley, C. K., Caez, H. J., and Mersheimer, W.: Primary bronchogenic carcinoma of the lung in children. Review of the literature; Report of a case. *AMA J. Dis. Child.* 82:49, 1951.
16. Hope, J. W. and Koop, C. E.: Differential diagnosis of mediastinal masses. *Ped. Clinics of N. A.* Vol. 6 2:379, May, 1959.
17. Bigelow, N. H., Klinger, S. and Wright, A. W.: Primary tumors of the heart in infancy and early childhood. *Cancer* 7:549, 1954.
18. Prichard, R. W.: Tumors of the heart. Review of the subject and report of one hundred and fifty cases. *AMA Arch. Path.* 51:98, 1951.
18a. Melicow, M. M. and Uson, A. C.: Palpable abdominal masses in infants and children: A report based on a review of 653 cases. *J. Urol.* 81:705, 1959.
19. Edmonson, H. A.: Differential diagnosis of tumors and tumor-like lesions of the liver in infancy and childhood. *AMA J. Dis. Child.* 91:168, 1956.
20. Roth, S. I. and Helwig, E. B.: Juvenile polyps of the colon and rectum. *Cancer* 16:468, 1963.
21. Mestel, A. L.: Lymphosarcoma of the small intestine in infancy and childhood. *Ann. Surg.* 149:87, 1959.
22. Wilcox, H. R., Jr. and Beattle, J. L.: Carcinoma complicating ulcerative colitis during childhood. *Am. J. Clin. Path.* 26:778, 1956.
23. Hempstead, R. H., Dockerty, M. B. Priestley, J. T. and Logan, G. B.: Hypernephroma in children. Report of two cases. *J. Urol.* 70:152, 1953.
24. Silva-Sosa, M., and Gonzalez-Cerna J.: Wilm's tumor in children; Review of 150 cases. *Prog. Clin. Cancer* 2:323, 1966.
25. Gross, R. C., Farber, S., and Martin, L. W.: Neuroblastoma sympatheticum. *Pediat.* 23:1179, 1959.
26. Horn, R. C., Jr. and Enterline, H. T.: Rhabdomyosarcoma: A clinicopathological study and classification of 39 cases. *Cancer* 11:181, 1958.
26a. Butt, J. A.: Ovarian tumors in childhood. *Am. J. Obst. & Gyn.* 69:833, 1955.
27. Dahlin, D. C.: *Bone Tumors.* Springfield, Illinois:Charles C Thomas, 1958.
28. Collins, V. P. and Collins, L. C.: Benign conditions simulating bone tumors, *JAMA* 160:431, 1956.
29. Kirkpatrick, J. A.: Tumors of the bone. *Ped. Clinics of N. A.* Vol. 6 2:557, May, 1959.

Roentgenographic Aspects of the Most Frequent Abdominal Malignancies in Children

Catherine A. Poole, M.D.

A variety of malignant lesions can occur in the abdomen during infancy and childhood, but certainly the majority prove ultimately to be either Wilms' tumor or neuroblastoma. In most cases either of these two masses can be defined in terms of origin and extent with routine diagnostic procedures including intravenous urography, and special procedures, such as angiography need not be utilized routinely in their preoperative evaluation.

The typical features of Wilms' tumor have been extensively reviewed. These are usually large flank masses, spherical in nature, often sharply demarcated, and oftentimes associated with haziness or obliteration of the ipsilateral psoas muscle. Calcification is infrequent in Wilms' tumor, occurring in approximately 10% or less. When calcification is present it can assume almost any appearance, though it is frequently curvilinear. The changes on intravenous urography are those of a large intrarenal parenchymal mass lesion, growing within a pseudocapsule produced by stretching and atrophy of the renal cortex on its expanding periphery. There is bizarre distortion of the pelvocalyceal system, which is elongated, stretched and displaced around the parenchymal mass (Fig. 1). Dilatation or amputation of calyces is common, and the ureter is displaced by the mass which commonly extends to the midline, and occasionally extends across the midline. The distortion will vary, depending upon where the bulk of the mass is in relationship to the pelvocalyceal system. The mass may be confined to one portion of the kidney, such as the lower pole or the lateral aspect (Fig. 2, A and B). On occasion the mass may diffusely infiltrate the entire kidney, and in this situation nonfunction of the kidney may occur.

Catherine A. Poole, M.D., *Associate Professor of Radiology and Pediatrics, Department of Radiology, University of Miami School of Medicine, Miami, Florida.*

*Portions of this article appeared originally in the American Journal of Roentgenology, Radium Therapy and Nuclear Medicine, Vol. C1X, No. 2, June, 1970, entitled, "Unusual Renal Masses in the Pediatric Age Group," by Catherine A. Poole, M.D., and Manuel Viamonte, Jr., M.D.

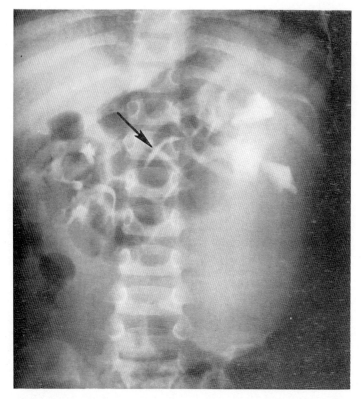

Fig. 1. Wilms' tumor. Bizarre distortion of the pelvocalyceal system is the typical change produced on intravenous urography by a large parenchymal Wilms' tumor. The pelvis is compressed and the ureter displaced cephalad and medially (arrow) by the bulk of the mass which extends across the midline.

Multiple views of the tumor should be obtained during intravenous urography. Prone, oblique, and lateral views are frequently more valuable than the routine supine views in the overall assessment of the lesion (Fig. 3, A and B). At least one of these views will usually demonstrate the typical displacement, elongation, and distortion of the pelvocalyceal system, and the pelvic and ureteral compression and displacement of Wilms' tumor (Fig. 4, A and B). These findings, though typical, are not specific, and obviously there is no radiographic finding which can substitute for a histologic diagnosis. From a practical standpoint, however, the odds are so overwhelming in favor of a mass of this nature being a Wilms' tumor that therapy is immediately instituted on that assumption.

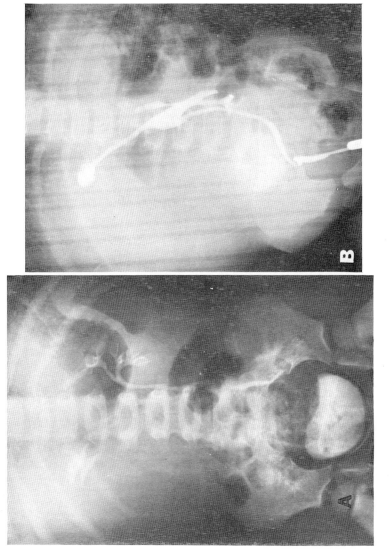

Fig. 2. Wilms' tumor. The distortion and displacement of the pelvocalyceal system and ureter by Wilms' tumor is dependent on the relationship of the bulk of the mass to these structures. A mass in the lower pole principally produces cephalad displacement (A), whereas a similar mass arising in the lateral aspect of the renal parenchyma produces prominent medial displacement (B), in addition to stretching and elongation.

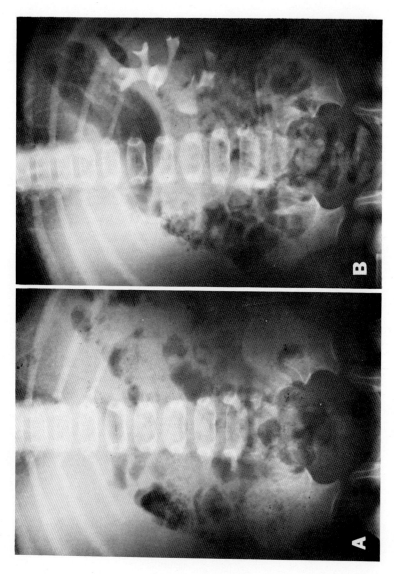

Fig. 3. Wilms' tumor. (A) A 12 cm hard palpable mass in the left flank of this 10 month old infant cannot be identified on a supine view of the abdomen. (B) Intravenous urography reveals enlargement of the left kidney with dilatation and slight distortion of the pelvocalyceal system. Neither the size nor the extent of the mass can be appreciated (Compare with Fig. 4).

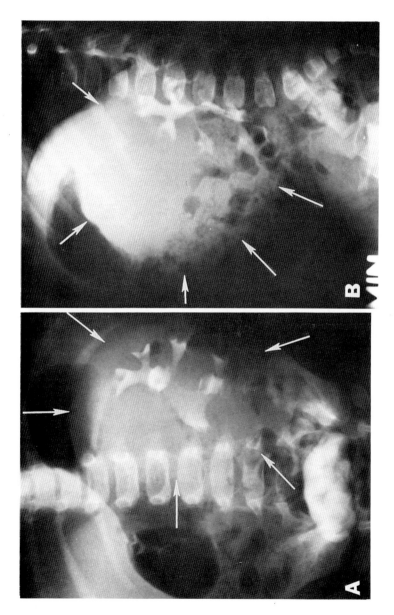

Fig. 4. Same case as Fig. 3. Prone (A) and lateral (B) views both demonstrate the size of the huge Wilms' tumor to better advantage than the supine views (Fig. 3), as well as the characteristic changes in the pelvocalyceal system produced by the parenchymal mass arising in the anterior aspect of the left kidney (arrows).

The only other preoperative study which must be obtained is the chest film, since up to thirty percent of patients with Wilms' tumor will have pulmonary metastases at the time of presentation. If the chest film is normal, it is perhaps not mandatory to obtain a routine skeletal survey. Skeletal metastases in Wilms' tumor are quite uncommon and when they do occur it is usually in the presence of disseminated disease elsewhere. In this situation, the chest film is almost inevitably positive, and a skeletal survey then does become mandatory.

The most common flank mass seen in infancy or childhood is of course, the hydronephrotic kidney. The radiographic findings in this situation depend upon the cause and the severity of the hydronephrosis. In the most severe cases, which are usually congenital ureteropelvic junction obstructions, renal function may be negligible and opacification will not be demonstrable on intravenous urography. In most cases, however, there is sufficient contrast material within the remaining compressed renal parenchyma that it can be seen outlining the hydronephrotic sac (Fig. 5A). Delayed roentgenograms will often reveal faint evidence of contrast material within a markedly dilated collecting system, sometimes taking as long as 24 hours to appear (Fig. 5B). The less severe forms of hydronephrosis are easily diagnosed by intravenous urography.

More common than Wilms' tumor in the neonatal age group is the unilateral multicystic kidney, the majority of these lesions being discovered within the first day or two of life. The avascular nature of these lesions can be demonstrated by the total body opacification effect during intravenous urography (Fig. 6). Total failure of excretory function will be evident, but on close inspection of the flank area the cysts can frequently be identified as round radiolucencies separated from each other by slightly opacified septa. This appearance of a flank mass is quite characteristic of a unilateral multicystic kidney, and should not be confused with Wilms' tumor which is rare in the neonatal age group. Confirmatory evidence can be obtained by filling the ureter in a retrograde fashion, demonstrating the ureteral atresia which is associated with the malformation of unilateral multicystic kidney.

These three lesions, then, Wilms' tumor, hydronephrosis, and unilateral multicystic kidney comprise the bulk of renal masses in infants and children. All three lesions have rather typical radiographic features which, when they are present, are extraordinarily accurate in defining the nature of the mass. Other intrarenal cystic and solid lesions, both benign and malignant, do occur in infants and children. Although uncommon, they should be considered in the differential diagnosis of a renal mass, particularly if the radiographic findings on intravenous urography are inconclusive. Renal angiography can contribute significant information in a situation of this nature. Nephrotomography has not proved useful in the evaluation of renal masses in this age group.

Differentiating extrarenal retroperitoneal masses from Wilms' tumor is not difficult in the majority of cases, and can usually be accomplished with routine

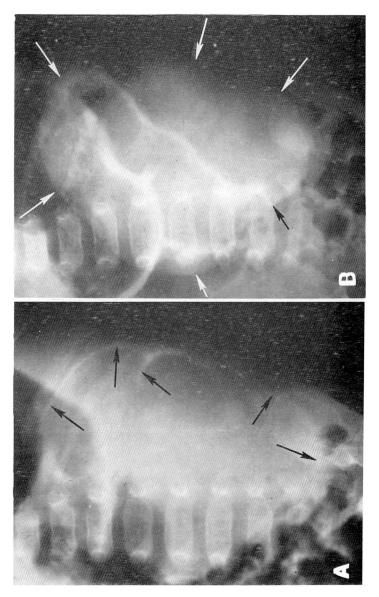

Fig. 5. Hydronephrosis. (A) Twenty minutes following its intravenous injection, contrast material opacifies compressed renal parenchyma (arrows) rimming a markedly dilated collecting system. (B) Twenty-four hour delayed roentgenogram demonstrates the contrast material diluted within the massively dilated pelvocalyceal system (arrows). The hydronephrosis is secondary to congenital ureteropelvic junction obstruction.

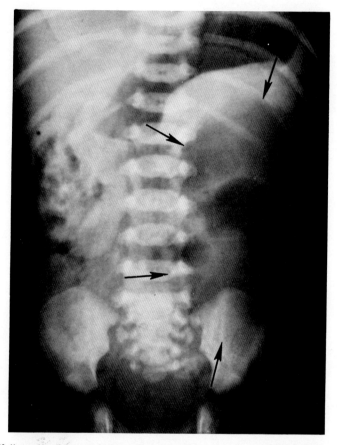

Fig. 6. Unilateral multicystic kidney. The avascular nature of unilateral multicystic kidney can be demonstrated during total body opacification by the large radiolucent area in the left flank (arrows). Compare to the normal nephrogram effect in the right kidney.

diagnostic procedures, including again, intravenous urography. The most common extrarenal malignancy occurring in the flank in infants and children is of course neuroblastoma. A flank mass can usually be identified on plain films of the abdomen. Neuroblastoma is typically an infiltrative lesion, it does not grow within a pseudocapsule as does Wilms' tumor, hence the mass usually lacks sharply defined margins. Calcification, which is rare in Wilms' tumor, is present in approximately 50% of (or more) neuroblastomas (Fig. 7). The calcification may be stippled, amorphous, linear, nodular, or rarely very dense and homogenous in appearance.

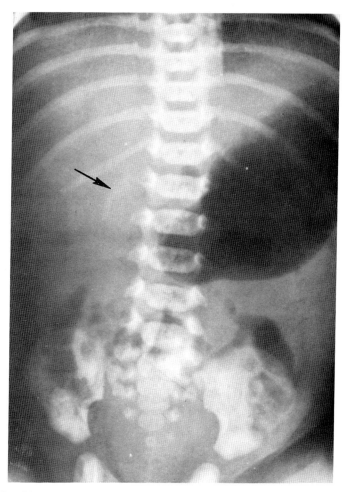

Fig. 7. Neuroblastoma. Calcification is present within a palpable mass in the right flank of a newborn infant (arrow). The mass was suprarenal on intravenous urography. Calcification is rare in Wilms' tumor which is seldom found in the new-born period.

The main differential features between Wilms' tumor and neuroblastoma are usually readily apparent on intravenous urography. Wilms', the intrarenal tumor, distorts, displaces, elongates and stretches the pelvocalyceal system. Neuroblastoma, the extrarenal tumor, will displace the kidney and rotate it on either its vertical or horizontal axis. The type of displacement and rotation encountered depends on the location of the bulk of the mass. The most common site of origin of neuroblastoma is the adrenal gland, in which case the kidney is displaced inferiorly and perhaps anteriorly, and at the same time is usually rotated anteriorly and laterally on its vertical axis (Fig. 8, A and B). Prone, oblique, and lateral views are frequently more helpful than the usual supine view in defining the type of renal displacement and rotation, and should be included as a routine part of the intravenous urogram in any infant or child with an abdominal mass.

The pelvocalyceal system is displaced and rotated with the kidney as a whole unit. Actual distortion of the pelvocalyceal system, as seen in Wilms' tumor, does not occur with neuroblastoma unless there is invasion of the kidney by the mass. Renal invasion by neuroblastoma to the point of producing pelvocalyceal distortion that may be confused with Wilms' tumor can occur, but has been distinctly uncommon in our series. In that situation, it may be difficult or impossible to distinguish the two lesions by intravenous urography, and in fact, it may be difficult to do so with angiography.

Less commonly neuroblastoma may arise outside the adrenal from any locale where neural crest tissue existed embryologically. Abdominal neuroblastoma can, therefore, originate anywhere from the level of the diaphragm down into the pelvis. They can arise medially to the kidney, displacing it laterally (Fig. 9). They can arise below the kidney, in which case it is the ureter which is displaced laterally. Or they can occur within the pelvis, in which case medial and anterior displacement of the bladder may be encountered.

It is unfortunate, that from 50 to as high as 90 percent of children with neuroblastoma have evidence of extension or spread of the lesion beyond the primary site at the time of presentation. Evidence of this extension or spread of neuroblastoma should be searched for in the abdomen, chest, and skeleton. In the abdomen involvement of retroperitoneal lymph nodes can be defined by the obstruction or displacement of the urinary tract which they frequently produce (Fig. 10). This involvement of the urinary tract can be seen ipsilateral or contralateral to the primary lesion. Obstruction or invasion of the kidney by a neuroblastoma severe enough to produce nonfunction on intravenous urography has been reported, but is quite unusual. In our experience a non-functioning malignant flank mass in a child is much more likely to be a Wilms' tumor than a neuroblastoma.

Approximately one half of our patients with neuroblastoma have shown evidence of paravertebral widening in the lower thoracic or upper lumbar area. This represents extension or spread up along the retroperitoneal lymph node chain (Fig. 11). This is not a specific finding for neuroblastoma, it can be found in other retroperitoneal lesions such as lymphoma or rhabdomyosarcoma. We have not identified this paravertebral widening in any of our patients with Wilms' tumor.

Pulmonary metastases which are common in Wilms' tumor are seldom identified in the chest film of a patient with neuroblastoma. Pleural metastases

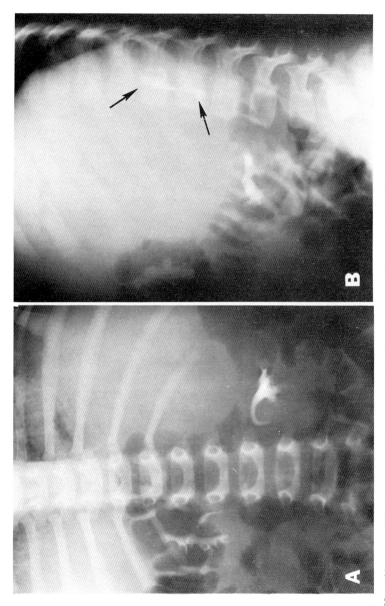

Fig. 8. Neuroblastoma. (A) A large neuroblastoma arising in the left adrenal displaces the left kidney inferiorly and rotates it laterally on its vertical axis. (B) Simultaneous anterior displacement and rotation of the left kidney is apparent on the lateral view, compared to the normal position of the right kidney (arrows). No distortion of the pelvocalyceal system is present.

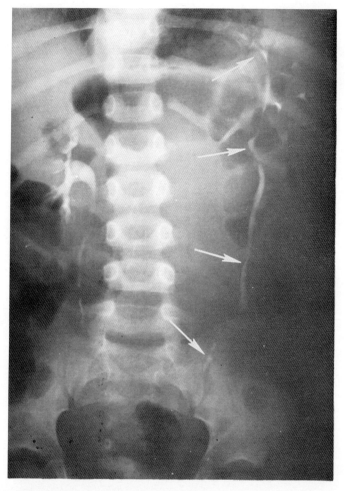

Fig. 9. Neuroblastoma. Large extra-adrenal neuroblastoma in the left retroperitoneal space displacing the left kidney laterally and slightly cephalad. The inferior aspect of the mass displaces the ureter laterally as far down as the pelvic brim (arrows). Slight distortion of the upper pelvocalyceal system suggests invasion of the upper pole of the left kidney.

on the other hand do occur in neuroblastoma, and can be associated with a very rapid accumulation of pleural fluid (Fig. 12, A and B).

Neuroblastoma, as opposed to Wilms' tumor, frequently metastasizes to bone, and it is not uncommon for these patients to present not because of an abdominal mass but because of symptoms related to this metastatic disease (Fig. 13, A and B). A skeletal survey is therefore mandatory in any child suspected of

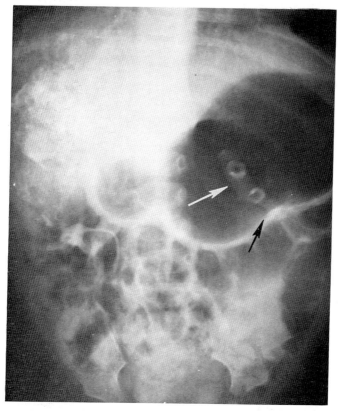

Fig. 10. Neuroblastoma. A large bulky calcified primary neuroblastoma in the right adrenal displaces and rotates the right kidney inferiorly and laterally. Extension or spread from the primary to lymph nodes in the hilum of the left kidney displaces that organ laterally and partially obstructs the pelvis and ureter with resultant hydronephrosis (arrows).

having neuroblastoma, which can metastasize literally to every bone in the body. The skull and facial bones, including the paranasal sinuses as well as all portions of the trunk and extremities should be scrutinized carefully for the presence of metastatic disease (Fig. 14, A and B). The lesions resemble those seen in children with leukemia, and their presence in the small bones of the hands or feet has been said to be a differential point in favor of leukemia as opposed to neuroblastoma. This has not been a valid observation in our experience, neuroblastoma and leukemia have involved the small bones of the hands and feet with equal frequency (Fig. 15). When bone lesions of this nature are discovered, a search should be undertaken in the abdomen, the chest, or perhaps even in the neck, to identify neuroblastoma as the potential primary lesion.

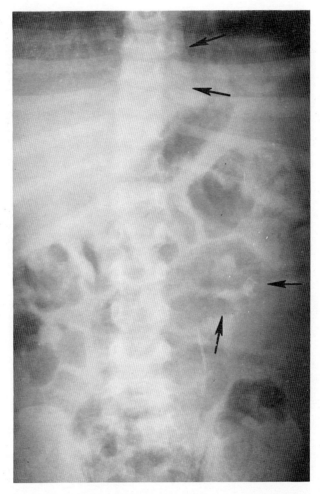

Fig. 11. Neuroblastoma. Paravertebral widening (upper arrows) is indicative of cephalad spread from a primary neuroblastoma in the left adrenal which displaces the left kidney inferiorly and rotates it laterally (lower arrows).

When a suprarenal lesion invades the upper pole of the kidney it may be impossible to identify the nature of the primary lesion with the usual diagnostic procedures. If the mass is in the right flank, it may even be impossible to exclude the possibility of a primary lesion in the liver. We have seen hepatoblastoma invading both the adrenal and the kidney, with metastatic disease to retro-peritoneal lymph nodes and to bone, mimicking neuroblastoma (Fig. 16).

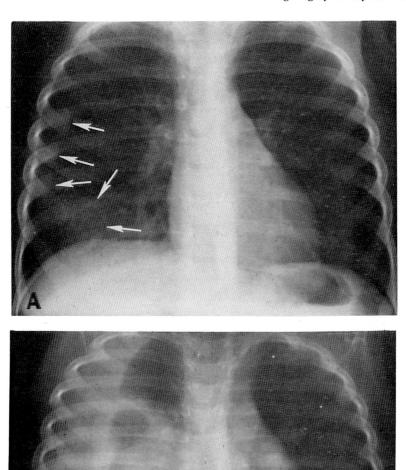

Fig. 12. Metastatic Neuroblastoma. (A) Metastatic pleural nodules from neuroblastoma (arrows), primary in the left adrenal (same patient as in Fig. 8, A and B). (B) Chest film two weeks later demonstrates the rapid accumulation of pleural fluid that may accompany metastatic pleural nodules.

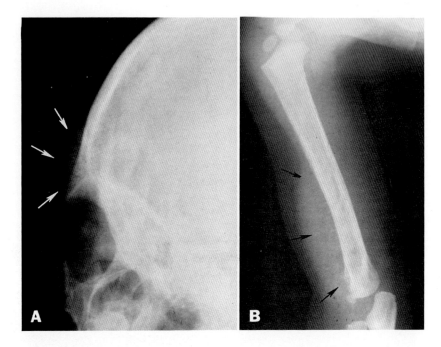

Fig. 13. Metastatic Neuroblastoma. (A) A two-year-old boy brought to the emergency room by the police, tentative diagnosis of a battered child because of a "black eye" and "bumps" on the forehead. The supraorbital lesion contained a "sunburst" spiculation of bone (arrows) indicating a malignant lesion. (B) A skeletal survey revealed a similar lesion in the right humerus. Intravenous urography revealed a primary suprarenal neuroblastoma.

Liver tumors can be recognized on plain films of the abdomen by the characteristic displacement of the gastrointestinal tract they produce, depending upon whether the bulk of the mass is in the right lobe, the left lobe, or whether it is a diffuse lesion throughout the liver. The urinary tract in this situation can either be normal, or the right kidney may show posterior and superior or inferior displacement on intravenous urography. Differentiation of the various types of intrahepatic tumors encountered in children is not possible with routine diagnostic studies. Occasionally the specific nature of the lesion can be suggested by the clinical presentation of the patient, such as an hemangioendothelioma of the liver in an infant, who presents with a classical clinical triad of hepatomegaly, cutaneous hemangiomas, and high output congestive heart failure. The pre-treatment evaluation of liver masses is nonetheless incomplete without angiography, which remains the best procedure currently available to define the nature of liver masses, their exact location, and to assess the feasibility of their surgical resection, which many of them are amenable to.

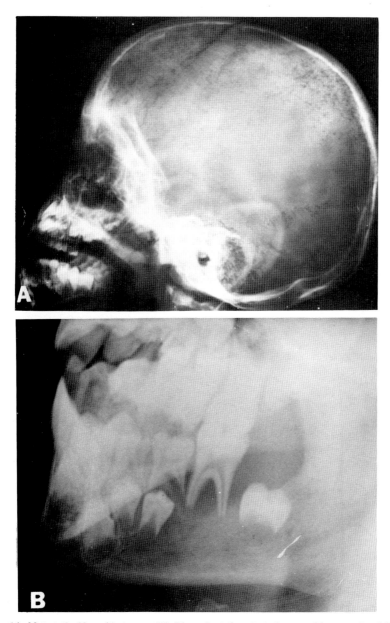

Fig. 14. Metastatic Neuroblastoma. (A) Disseminated metastatic neuroblastoma involving the cranial vault, base of the skull and facial bones. The cranial sutures are not separated, as frequently occurs in this situation. (B) Metastatic neuroblastoma involving the mandible with loss of alveolar bone, lamina dura, dental follicles, and resorption of root tips. "Floating teeth" of this nature are identical to those found in histiocytoses.

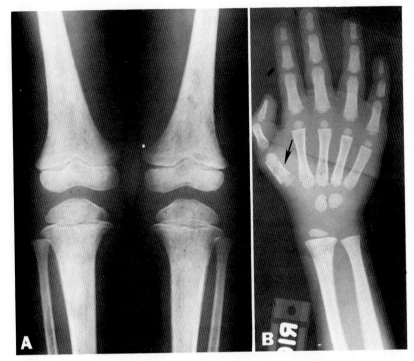

Fig. 15. Metastatic Neuroblastoma. (A) Diffuse lytic lesions with associated periosteal elevation are similar radiographically to bone lesions that might be seen in leukemia and other metastatic malignancies. Intravenous urography revealed a primary neuroblastoma in the right adrenal. (B) Metastatic neuroblastoma can involve the small bones of the hands (arrow) or feet similar to leukemia. The distal radius is also involved with metastatic neuroblastoma.

Summary

The majority of abdominal masses in infants and children are renal and suprarenal in origin. The most common suprarenal mass is, of course, neuroblastoma. Hydronephrosis, unilateral multicystic kidney, and Wilms' tumor comprise the bulk of renal masses seen in this age group. In the majority of cases, these lesions can be identified with a high degree of accuracy utilizing intravenous urography in conjunction with routine films of the chest, abdomen and skeleton. Use of special procedures in abdominal masses with typical radiographic features need not be routine, but rather can be limited to those cases in which the routine procedures lead to inconclusive results in terms of diagnosis or treatment planning. The only masses in which special procedures, specifically angiography, are routinely employed in pre-treatment evaluation are

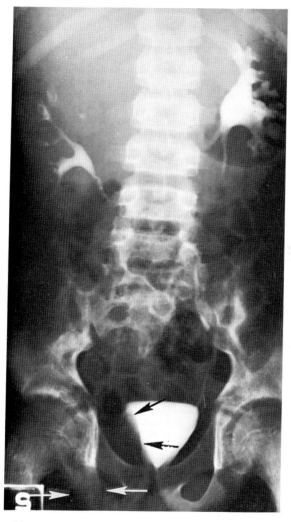

Fig. 16. Hepatoblastoma. A noncalcified mass in the right upper quadrant could be a primary renal mass because of the distortion of the upper collecting system, or a suprarenal mass with invasion of the upper pole. Evidence of metastatic spread to pelvic nodes displacing the bladder (black arrows) as well as to bone (white arrows) favored the diagnosis of neuroblastoma. A biopsy of the ischial bone lesion was felt to be compatible with neuroblastoma. The patient later expired, final autopsy diagnosis was hepatoblastoma which had invaded both the right adrenal and kidney with disseminated lymphatic and bony metastases.

those involving the liver. Selective angiography remains the best method currently available for obtaining information regarding not only the specific nature of liver masses, but outlining their vascular anatomy, knowledge of which is essential prior to operative intervention if such is feasible.

References

1. Black, W. C. and Ragsdale, E. F.: Wilms' tumor, *Amer. J. Roentgen.* 103:53-60, 1968.
2. Eklof, O. and Gooding, Ch. A.: Paravertebral widening in cases of neuroblastoma. *Brit. J. Radiol.* 40:358-365, 1967.
3. Eklof, O. and Lundin, E.: Renal pelvis appearances in nephro and neuroblastoma. *Acta Radiologica* (Diagnosis) 8:209-220, 1969.
4. Favara, B. E., Johnson, W., and Ito, J.: Renal tumors in neonatal period. *Cancer* 22:845-855, 1968.
5. Gleason, D. G., McAlister, W. H., and Kissane, J.: Cystic disease of kidneys in children. *Amer. J. Roentgen.* 100:135-146, 1967.
6. Griscom, N. T.: Roentgenology of neonatal abdominal masses. *Amer. J. Roentgen.* 93:437-463, 1965.
7. Hope, J. W., and Borns, P. F.: Radiologic diagnosis of primary and metastatic cancer in infants and children. *Radiological Clin. N. Amer.* 3:353-374, 1965.
8. Hope, J. W., Borns, P. F., and Koop, C. E.: Diagnosis and treatment of neuroblastoma and embroma of the kidney. *Radiological Clin. N. Amer.* 1:593-619, 1963.
9. Karafin, L., Kirkpatrick, J. A., and Livingston, W. O.: Non-visualization of the kidney by excretory urography associated with neoplastic retroperitoneal masses in infants and children. *Journal of Urology.* 88: 459-463, 1962.
10. Lalli, A. F., Ahstrom, L., and Ericsson, N. O., and Rudhe, U.: Nephroblastoma (Wilms' tumor): urographic diagnosis and prognosis, *Radiology,* 87:495-500, 1966.
11. O'Connor, J. F., and Neuhauser, E. B. D.: Total body opacification in conventional and high dose intravenous urography in infancy. *Amer. J. Roentgen.* 90: 63-71, 1963.
12. Poole, C. A., and Viamonte, M., Jr:, Unusual renal masses in the pediatric age group. *Amer. J. Roentgen.* 109: 368-379, 1970.
13. Poole, C. A., Keusch, K. D., and King, D. R.: The significance of "floating teeth" in children. *Radiology,* 86: 215-219, 1966.

Special Procedures in Roentgen Diagnosis of Abdominal Tumors in Infancy and Childhood

Catherine A. Poole, M.D.

Special procedures, specifically angiography, are not utilized routinely in the evaluation of abdominal masses in infants and children. Hydronephrosis, unilateral multicystic kidney, and Wilms' tumor compromise the bulk of renal masses seen in this age group, whereas neuroblastoma is the most frequent extrarenal lesion encountered. Intravenous urography has proven to be an accurate study, leading to the correct preoperative diagnosis in the vast majority of these lesions. If typical radiographic features of these lesions are defined by intravenous urography, therapy is ordinarily instituted without further radiographic work-up other than for a chest film and skeletal survey.

A procedure that has been recommended as routine because of its simplicity is an inferior venacavogram. This is not a special procedure per se, but entails utilizing a leg vein to inject a bolus of contrast material and visualizing the inferior vena cava by early filming during the routine intravenous urogram. There are several problems inherent in the interpretation of inferior venacavograms performed in this manner that limit the usefulness of the examination. Any large mass which is adjacent to it can displace the inferior vena cava, whether the mass is benign or malignant. Faint visualization or even complete non-visualization of the inferior vena cava, with shunting through the pelvic veins to the rich retroperitoneal ascending lumbar collateral channels to the azygous system, does not imply that the inferior vena cava is invaded or totally obstructed (Fig. 1). The inferior vena cava may be merely displaced or partially compressed, and rarely even a vigorous Valsalva maneuver can produce this same phenomena in the absence of a mass. Normal streaming can sometimes be

Catherine A. Poole, M.D., *Associate Professor of Radiology and Pediatrics, Department of Radiology, University of Miami School of Medicine, Miami, Fla.*

*Portions of this article appeared originally in the *American Journal of Roentgenology, Radium Therapy and Nuclear Medicine,* Volume C1X, Number 2, June, 1970, entitled, "Unusual Renal Masses in the Pediatric Age Group," by Catherine A. Poole, M.D. and Manuel Viamonte Jr., M.D.

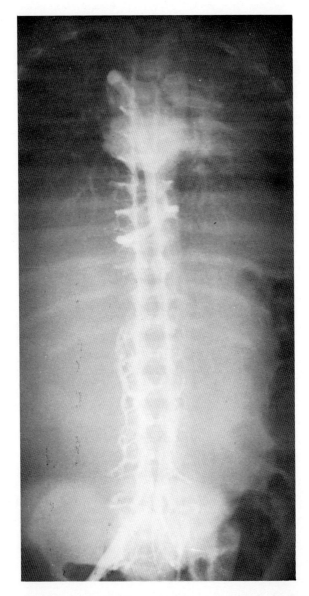

Fig. 1. Inferior Venacavogram. Ten-month-old infant with massive right Wilms' tumor. Peripheral venacavography reveals non-visualization of the vena cava with shunting through lumbar collateral channels to the azygous system. The vena cava was not invaded at surgery, but rather externally compressed by the bulk of the mass.

confused with involvement by invasion of the inferior vena cava when the examination is performed in this manner.

To be of more value, the inferior venacavogram should be performed utilizing the catheter technique, with biplane multiple filming. At that point it would cease to be considered a routine procedure. Even done in this manner the inferior venacavogram is of limited value. The limits of the mass may be defined, but the examination offers no information as to the origin or the nature of the mass. Compression or actual invasion of the inferior vena cava can be demonstrated by this technique, but this finding does not imply that the lesion is unresectable. This is particularly true in children with Wilms' tumor. For these reasons, inferior venacavography is seldom used in infants or children with abdominal masses, and we do not feel it is indicated as a routine procedure.

Lymphangiography is no longer utilized as a routine procedure in children with solid mass lesions. In relative value the procedure has not proven profitable in terms of information gained. Lymphangiography in infants and children is now limited primarily to the staging of lymphomas, or to the evaluation of retroperitoneal masses which we have not been able to define by other methods. In these situations lymphangiography has proven quite useful.

Angiography, on the other hand, has proven to be an excellent diagnostic tool, which can frequently provide information otherwise unobtainable by methods short of surgery. The indications for angiography vary, but in general it can be utilized in any situation in which the diagnosis, extent, or the management of the mass lesion is in question.

Renal Masses

The largest group of infants and children in whom special procedures have been utilized in the evaluation of abdominal masses are those with unusual renal lesions. Some of the indications for performing aortography and renal angiography, and the benefit to be gained from these procedures are outlined in the following case reports.

Case 1:

A. F., a 16-year-old boy, was evaluated because of the recent onset of hematuria. Physical examination on admission was negative, an abdominal mass was not palpable. A benign cyst in the upper pole of the right kidney was suggested on intravenous urography, which included tomography. Renal angiography confirmed the presence of a vascular mass within the upper pole of the right kidney, with neovascularity consistent with a malignant lesion, most likely Wilms' tumor (Fig. 2, A and B). A chest film revealed three metastatic nodules in the left lower lobe, a skeletal survey revealed no evidence of metastatic disease to bone. A right nephrectomy was performed, and histologic findings confirmed the diagnosis of Wilms' tumor.

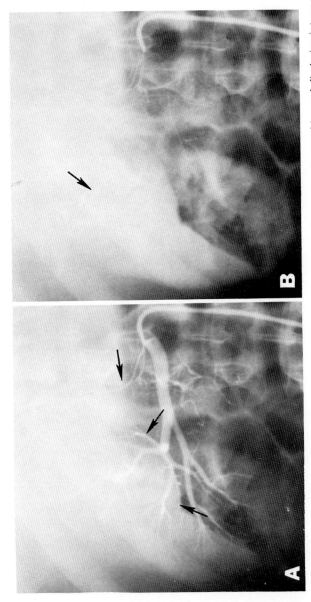

Fig. 2. Case 1. Wilms' tumor. (**A**) Selective right renal angiography reveals a mass in the upper pole stretching and displacing intrarenal and capsular branches (*arrows*). Neovascularity is present within the mass. (**B**) Nephrogram phase reveals replacement of renal parenchyma, an irregular, inhomogeneous nephrogram and stasis in vessels (*arrow*).

Comment: The unusual occurrence of renal masses, benign or malignant, in this age group prompted renal angiography. Displacement, stretching and attenuation of both intrarenal and capsular branches of the right renal artery confirmed the location of the mass within the right upper pole. Neovascularity was present within the mass. These pathologic vessels are characterized by their abnormal appearance, number, distribution and branching pattern. They lack normal tapering, are pleomorphic, and exhibit unusual tortuosity (Fig. 2A). The nephrographic phase demonstrated compression and replacement of renal substance by tumor tissue, stasis of contrast material in arteries, and apparent early venous return (Fig. 2B). These findings are similar to those described with Wilms' tumor. Pooling or laking, and marked hypervascularity and arteriovenous shunting seen frequently in renal cell carcinoma are usually not seen in Wilms' tumor.

Case 2:

L. B., a 5-year-old girl, was evaluated for what was clinically felt to be an enlarged spleen, discovered on a routine preschool examination. The mother had been informed of the mass two years previously, and was told that the child had "kissing disease." Intravenous urography revealed posterior displacement and compression of the left collecting system by a large mass in the anterior aspect of the left kidney (Fig. 3, A and B). Wilms' tumor was felt to be unlikely in view of the history, and in the absence of any gross distortion of the collecting system. Renal angiography confirmed the intrarenal location of the mass, by marked stretching of the intrarenal arteries over the circumference of the mass. The lesion was totally avascular and the compression of the renal parenchyma bordering the mass indicated that it was a large benign cortical renal cyst (Fig. 4). Wilms' tumor has been reported occurring in the wall of a large solitary cyst, or in association with multiple cysts in one kidney, but there is no evidence of such in this case. At surgery a benign cortical renal cyst was removed, the left kidney was conserved.

Comment: Angiography is of value when the site of origin or the nature of a mass lesion is uncertain. Simple renal cysts, although common in adults, are quite rare in children. The most important entity to differentiate from a simple renal cyst in this age group is Wilms' tumor, and the two lesions may be indistinguishable by routine intravenous urography. Angiography can usually differentiate a benign cystic lesion from Wilms' tumor which virtually always shows some degree of neovascularity. Nephrotomography has not proved useful in this regard in young patients.

Case 3:

J. A. was 11 years old when he presented with left flank pain and hematuria of two weeks' duration. Intravenous urography revealed enlargement of the left kidney with diminution of function as compared to the right kidney which was

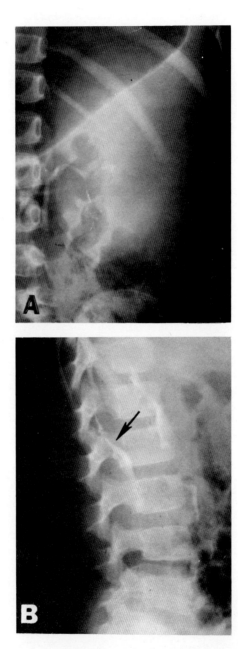

Fig. 3. Case 2. Renal Cyst. **(A)** A large mass in the left flank is compressing the collecting system of the left kidney from which it cannot be separated. **(B)** The left collecting system is displaced posteriorly (*arrow*) but is not otherwise distorted.

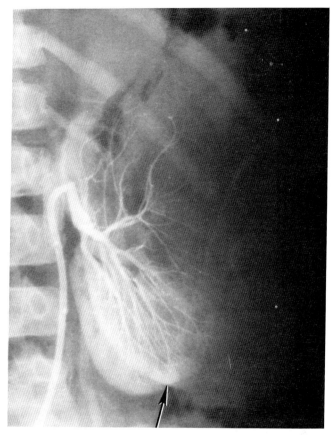

Fig. 4. Same case as in Fig. 3, **A** and **B**. Selective left renal angiography reveals stretching and displacement of intrarenal branches over the circumference of a totally avascular mass. Localized compression of renal parenchyma over the edge of the avascular lesion (*arrow*) is typical of a large renal cyst.

normal. Stretching and narrowing of the pelvocalyceal system suggested polycystic disease, which was felt to be unlikely because the changes were not bilateral (Fig. 5). Renal vein thrombosis and the rare Wilms' tumor which may diffusely infiltrate the kidney could produce similar changes. The distinction of these two lesions is important because non-surgical conservative management of the former is frequently possible.

Stretching and straightening of otherwise normal intrarenal arteries was demonstrated by angiography (Fig. 6A). Diminished blood flow was evidenced by the poor and delayed nephrogram effect, and at no time was the renal vein visualized (Fig. 6B). There was no evidence of neovascularity or tumor

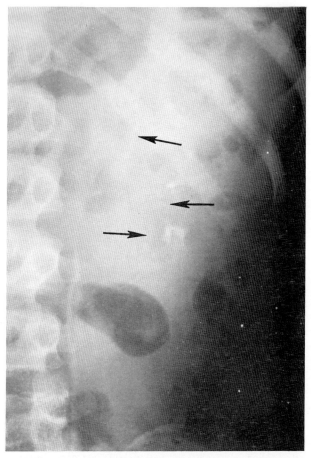

Fig. 5. Case 3. Renal Vein Thrombosis. The left kidney is enlarged and function is diminished. The calyces and infundibulae are stretched and narrowed (*arrows*). The right kidney was normal.

replacement of renal parenchyma. A diagnosis of renal vein thrombosis was thereby suggested, and malignancy as the underlying etiology excluded.

Comment: Angiography can provide valuable information regarding renal masses that may otherwise be unobtainable by methods short of surgery. This information is particularly valuable when conservative non-surgical management of the patient may be indicated. Arteriography and/or retrograde renal venography can be useful in establishing a diagnosis of renal vein thrombosis, and excluding malignancy as a predisposing cause which must always be considered in an older child or adult with that diagnosis.

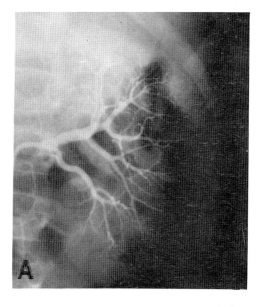

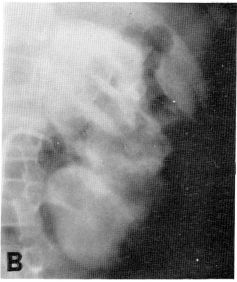

Fig. 6. Same case as in Fig. 5. (A) Selective left renal angiogram reveals slight stretching and straightening of interlobar branches, with no evidence of neovascularity. (B) A poor and delayed nephrogram is still evident at 16 seconds. The left renal vein was never visualized.

Case 4:

W. S., a 6-year-old boy, was admitted with the diagnosis of acute glomerulonephritis. Intravenous urography revealed a normal left kidney, and suggested the possibility of a mass in the right kidney (Fig. 7). Nephrotomography suggested that the area in question was not avascular. Renal angiography revealed no evidence of stretching or displacement of intrarenal branches, and no evidence of neovascularity. The area in question was totally avascular, without the appearance of a space-occupying lesion (Fig. 8A). Aortography confirmed that the area in question was normal renal tissue supplied by an accessory renal artery (Fig. 8B). The finding was a normal variant.

Comment: Accessory renal arteries, polar hypertrophy, or persistent fetal lobulation are some examples of normal anatomic variations which may mimic neoplasia on intravenous urography. Angiography can exclude neoplasia in these situations, by the demonstration of normal vascular and nephrogram phases.

Case 5:

G. L. was born with a palpable mass in the right flank. In view of unrelated medical problems it was felt that surgery should be postponed if it was at all safe to do so. Aortography was performed by way of an umbilical catheter which was in place in the lower dorsal aorta. The left renal artery and the vascularity of the left kidney was normal. There was no evidence of a right renal artery (Fig. 9). The nephrographic phase revealed a normal nephrogram on the left, no

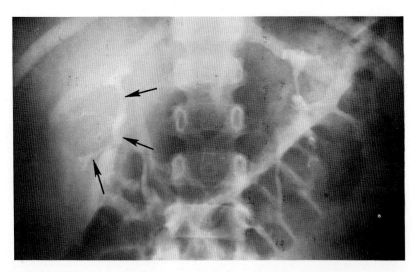

Fig. 7. Case 4. Pseudotumor. Intravenous urography suggests the possibility of a mass in the mid portion of the right kidney (*arrows*) displacing calyces and infundibula. The left kidney is normal.

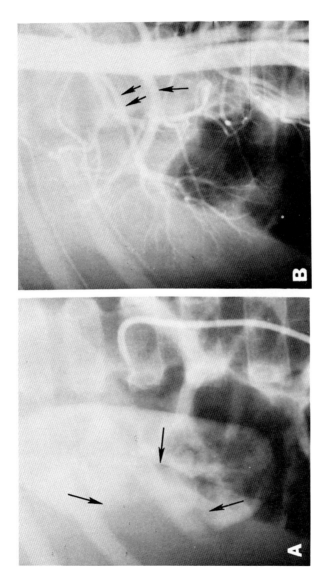

Fig. 8. Same case as Fig. 7. (A) Selective injection of the main right renal artery revealed no displacement of interlobar branches or neovascularity. The area in question on the intravenous urogram (*arrows*) is totally avascular and not a space occupying lesion. (B) Aortography reveals an accessory renal artery (*double arrows*) arising above the main renal artery (*single arrow*) supplying normal renal tissue.

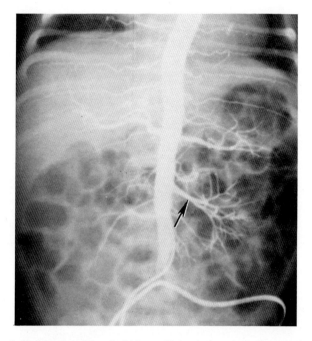

Fig. 9. Case 5. Unilateral multicystic kidney. Abdominal aortography reveals a normal left renal artery (*arrow*), with no evidence of a right renal artery. The other major branches of the aorta are normal.

nephrogram on the right. A postangiographic view of the abdomen revealed a normal kidney on the left, with no evidence of renal function on the right. The mass was felt to represent a unilateral multicystic kidney, and that surgery could be safely postponed. A unilateral multicystic kidney was subsequently removed at the age of three months.

Comment: Unilateral multicystic kidney is a common flank mass in the neonatal age group, the majority of these lesions being discovered within the first day or two of life. These lesions are avascular, the associated renal artery being very small or completely absent. Total failure of excretory function will be evident on intravenous urography. A hydronephrotic kidney is not associated with absence of the renal artery. The intrarenal branches will be thinned, stretched and attenuated, depending on the severity of the hydronephrosis, they show no evidence of neovascularity. Wilms' tumor is rare in this age group, but neuroblastoma occasionally occurs in the neonate. Neither of these lesions is associated with absence of the renal artery, and neovascularity is virtually always present.

Case 6:

W. J. was a 2-year-old boy whose abdominal mass was known to have been present for at least four months according to his mother. The clinical impression was that of a typical Wilms' tumor in the right flank. Intravenous urography demonstrated a large mass lesion probably arising from the inferior pole of the right kidney, with the bulk of the mass projecting exorenally (Fig. 10). Aortography and angiography demonstrated the typical features of Wilms' tumor. The aorta and its branches were displaced by the bulk of the mass. The right renal artery was elevated and elongated, and displacement of the capsular and intrarenal branches confirmed the lower pole locale of the mass. Prominent neovascularity was present within the mass. The appearance, number, distribution and branching pattern of the vessels were abnormal. They lacked normal tapering, were pleomorphic, and exhibited unusual tortuosity and showed many small focal areas of dilatation suggestive of microaneurysm formation (Fig. 11A). The nephrographic phase demonstrated compression and replacement of renal substance by tumor tissue, stasis of contrast material within the arteries, and early venous return (Fig. 11B).

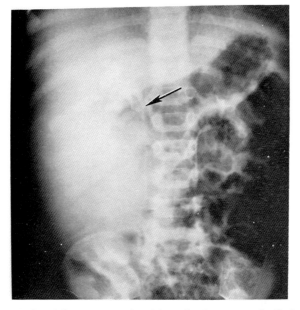

Fig. 10. Case 6. Renal hamartoma. The right collecting system is displaced medially, cephalad, and posteriorly by a large mass arising in the lower pole of the right kidney. The pelvis is elevated and compressed but the ureter is not displaced (*arrow*) by the large mass despite its extension to the midline.

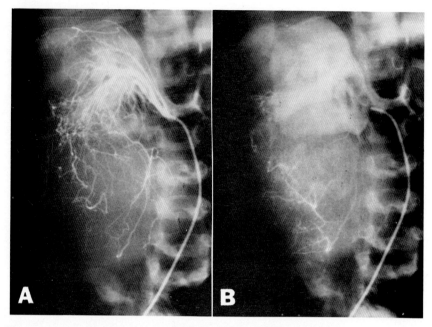

Fig. 11. Same case as Fig. 10. (A) Selective right renal angiography confirms the presence of a large mass within the lower pole of the right kidney. Abundant neovascularity within the mass is quite typical of that associated with Wilms' tumor. (B) The nephrogram phase demonstrates replacement of renal parenchyma, an irregular inhomogenous nephrogram and stasis in some arteries.

At surgery the bulk of the mass was extrarenal from its origin within the lower pole. It was a well encapsulated mass, and the cut surface was smooth, hard and white with a whorled strand pattern. The histologic sections showed the lesion to be composed of fairly uniform spindle cells forming a mixture of mature and immature fibrous tissue in interlacing bundles. No tubular or other epithelial elements or smooth or striated muscle or other mesenchymal elements were identified. The final pathologic diagnosis was that of a mesenchymal tumor, or fibrous hamartoma.

Comment: The hamartoma is one of a variety of pseudoneoplasias which have been encountered both in adults and in children. Neovascularity, though highly suggestive, is not specific for malignancy. False positive epinephrine tests have been described with renal hamartoma. We have observed false positive and false negative epinephrine tests. We have also seen one example of xanthogranulomatous pyelonephritis in a child which at angiography showed evidence of neovascularity, extension beyond the capsule, renal vein thrombosis with collateral circulation, and a false positive epinephrine test. Continual emphasis must be placed on the fact that no radiographic finding can substitute for a histologic diagnosis of malignancy. The significance of this becomes paramount when a therapeutic regimen of preoperative irradiation without histologic confirmation is contemplated in a patient with "typical" clinical, radiographic, and angiographic features of Wilms' tumor.

Liver Masses

Liver masses constitute one group of abdominal masses in infants and children in which special procedures, angiography and radioisotope scanning techniques, must be utilized routinely in pretreatment planning. Angiography is currently the best method available for determining the location, extent, and nature of hepatic masses, and to assess the feasibility of surgical resection which many of them are amenable to.

The most common primary malignant tumor of the liver in children is the hepatoma. This is the fourth commonest intra-abdominal malignancy in children, following Wilms', neuroblastoma, and rhabdomyosarcoma, and it is the commonest carcinoma encountered in this age group. These tumors tend to be multinodular, and confined to one lobe of the liver, the right more than the left, in which case the mass may be resectable. Uncommonly hepatoma may diffusely involve the entire liver.

The vascular supply to hepatomas is derived almost exclusively from the hepatic arterial system, and these lesions are best studied by selective celiac or hepatic angiography. The hepatoma, because of its tremendous functional demand is characterized by very large feeding vessels. The intrahepatic branches are widened, displaced, and stretched. There are numerous large, irregular, bizarre tumor vessels within these vascular masses. A dense tumor stain will persist for up to ten seconds or more, but large sinusoidal spaces or pools are not identified. Displacement and/or thrombosis of the portal vein will usually be evident if it is visualized.

The importance of angiography in the evaluation of liver masses is exemplified in the following case reports.

Case 7:

G. H. was 36 hours of age when she was admitted with the diagnosis of a mass in the left lobe of the liver. The mass was firm to palpation, there was no evidence of cutaneous hemangiomata, and the patient was not in congestive heart failure. Angiography revealed a large mass seemingly occupying the entire left lobe of the liver, fed by a very large left hepatic artery. The tumor was highly vascular, individual vessels were stretched and displaced, and tumor vascularity simulated (Fig. 12, A and B). Other features were present that characterized the lesion as a hemangioma as opposed to hepatoma. The feeding vessels were somewhat smaller than those noted in hepatomas, and they filled

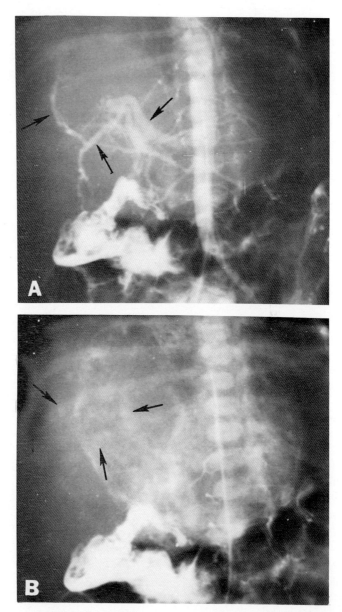

Fig. 12. Case 7. Cavernous hemangioma of the liver. (A) Aortography reveals a very large hepatic artery and feeding vessels (*arrows*) supplying a highly vascular mass occupying the left lobe of the liver. Individual vessels are stretched and displaced, and neovascularity is apparent. (B) Contrast material fills multiple well defined sinusoidal spaces (*arrows*) but arteriovenous shunting is not apparent.

large irregular well defined sinusoidal spaces which have been shown to retain contrast material for up to twenty seconds or longer. The portal vein was neither displaced nor thrombosed. Massive shunting with early appearance of venous structures is another characteristic feature of hemangiomas, which was not evident in this case. At surgery a large cavernous hemangioma occupying the left lobe of the liver was successfully resected.

Comment: Hemangiomas are the most common benign masses encountered in the liver of infants and children. Two types are encountered, cavernous and capillary, the latter of which is often associated with cutaneous hemangiomas. The capillary hemangioma is by far the more common in children and occurs almost exclusively in the first six months of life. These lesions are more commonly referred to as infantile hemangioendotheliomas because of their pronounced cellularity. Either type of hemangioma is amenable to surgical resection if confined to one lobe of the liver. Frequently they occur diffusely throughout the liver and are not amenable to surgical resection. Angiography plays a major role in this determination.

Case 8:

A. L. presented at 18-months-of-age with a large cystic mass in the right upper quadrant. Radiographic examination of the urinary and gastrointestinal tracts suggested that the mass was in the right lobe of the liver. A liver scan suggested that the mass was extrinsic to the liver, so angiography was undertaken to determine the site of origin and the nature of the mass. Angiography revealed displacement of the celiac axis and the right and left hepatic arteries, with no large feeding vessels (Fig. 13A). Close inspection of the branches of the right hepatic artery revealed that they were markedly stretched and attenuated over the rim of a large and totally avascular mass on the periphery of the right lobe. A large cystic lesion was surgically resected from the right lobe of the liver, which histologically showed evidence of connective tissue, bile ducts and liver cells with overgrowth of mesenchymal elements and degeneration of connective tissue with fluid collection within pseudocysts. The lesion was a benign mesenchymal hamartoma of the liver.

Comment: Hamartomas of the liver vary in the amount of vascular tissue which they contain. Some hamartomas are cystic in nature and totally avascular as this lesion was. Others appear vascular in nature, and simulate malignancy on angiography.

Case 9:

M. P., a 21-year-old woman, presented at another hospital with the sudden onset of severe abdominal pain. The patient was explored with the preoperative diagnosis of a possible ruptured viscus. A very large "placenta-like" mass was encountered in the right upper quadrant. The mass was biopsied, and the patient

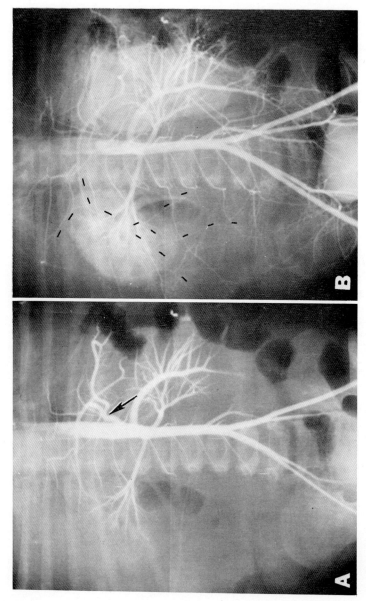

Fig. 13. Cystic hamartoma of the liver. **(A)** Abdominal aortography reveals displacement of the coelia axis and its branches superiorly and to the left (*arrow*). The right renal artery is stretched and straightened but there is no evidence of an intrarenal mass. **(B)** Branches of the right hepatic artery (*dotted lines*) are markedly stretched and attenuated over the circumference of a large and totally avascular mass on the periphery of the right lobe of the liver.

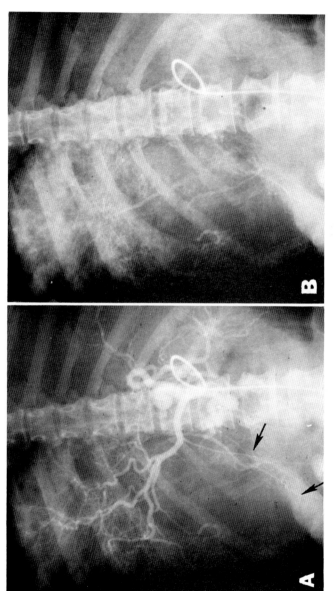

Fig. 14. Vascular hamartoma of the liver. (A) Selective hepatic angiography reveals stretching and displacement of numerous large and tortuous vessels occupying virtually the entire liver. Neovascularity is apparent throughout almost the entire liver except for an avascular area on the periphery of the right lobe (*arrows*) suggesting hemorrhage or necrosis. (B) A very dense, prolonged, irregular tumor stain, and vascular stasis is evident in the hepatogram phase.

was subsequently referred for further evaluation Angiography revealed a huge mass involving virtually the entire liver. The mass was very vascular, with displacement and stretching of numerous tortuous vessels (Fig. 14, A and B). A very dense, prolonged, irregular tumor stain was present, with a large avascular area on the periphery of the right lobe suggesting necrosis or hemorrhage. The angiographic diagnosis was hepatoma, diffuse and unresectable. The biopsy was that of a benign hamartoma.

Comment: Vascular hamartomas of the liver can mimic malignancy, just as those of the kidney can mimic malignancy of that organ. This reemphasizes the nonspecificity of neovascularity.

Summary

Angiography is a valuable adjunct in the preoperative evaluation of abdominal masses in infants and children. The indications for angiography vary; it is not used routinely with the exception of mass lesions involving the liver. Valuable information can be obtained regarding the origin and extent of the mass in question, as well as to the nature of the mass. Angiographic changes are not specific however, both false positive and false negative results have been obtained. There are no radiographic criteria by which one can make a histologic diagnosis.

Acknowledgement

The author expresses appreciation to James R. Le Page, M.D., Assistant Professor of Radiology and Chief, Division of Cardiac and Vascular Radiology, University of Miami School of Medicine, and to the Senior Fellows in Cardiovascular Radiology, whose contributions made this manuscript possible.

References

1. Abrams, R. M., Beranbaum, E. R., Santos, J. S., Lipson, J.: Angiographic features of cavernous hemangioma of the liver. *Radiology,* 92:308-312, 1969.
2. Becker, J. A., Fleming, R., Kanter, I. and Melicow, M.: Misleading appearances in renal angiography. *Radiology* 88:691-700, 1967.
3. Berdon, W. E., Baker, D. H.: Giant hepatic hemangioma with cardiac failure in the newborn period. *Radiology* 92:1523-1528, 1969.
4. Brinsfield, D., Blank, J. W., Sybers, R. G.: Aortography in children with abdominal masses. *J. Pediat.* 73:203-211, 1968.
5. Clark, R. E., Moss, A. A., DeLorimier, A. A., and Palubinskas, A.J.: Arteriography of Wilms' tumor. *Amer. J. Roentgen.* 113:476-490, 1971.
6. Dautrebande, J., Duckett, G., and Roy, P.: Claw sign and cortical cyst in renal angiography. *J. of Canad. Assoc. of Radiol.* 18:240-250, 1967.
7. Farah, J., Lofstrom, J. E.: Angiography of Wilms' tumor. *Radiology* 90:775-777, 1968.
8. Felson, B., and Moskowitz, M.: Renal pseudotumors: The regenerated nodule and other lumps, bumps, and dromedary humps. *Amer. J. Roentgen.* 107:720-729, 1969.

9. Folin, J.: Angiography in Wilms' tumour. *Acta Radiologica* (Diagnosis) 8:201-208, 1969.
10. Fredens, M.: Angiography in primary hepatic tumours in children. *Acta Radiologica* (Diagnosis) 8:193-200, 1969.
11. Gammill, S. L., Takahashi, M., Kawanami, M., Font, R., and Sparks, R.: Hepatic angiography in the selection of patients with hepatomas for hepatic lobectomy. *Radiology* 101:549-554, 1971.
12. Gyepes, M. T., and Burko, H.: Diffuse bilateral Wilms' tumor simulating multicystic renal disease. *Radiology* 82:1029-1031, 1964.
13. Harrell, J. E., Reeder, M. M., McAllister, H. A.: Case of the month from the A.F.I.P.: Exercise in radiologic-pathologic correlation. *Radiology* 91:1226-1232, 1968.
14. Koehler, P. R., Bowles, W. T., and McAllister, W. H.: Renal arteriography in experimental renal vein occlusion. *Radiology* 86: 851-855, 1966.
15. Meany, T. F.: Errors in angiographic diagnosis of renal masses. *Radiology* 93:361-366, 1969.
16. Meng, C. H., and Elkin, M.: Angiographic manifestations of Wilms' tumor: Observation of six cases. *Amer. J. Roentgenol.* 105:95-104, 1969.
17. McDonald, P.: Hepatic tumors in childhood. *Clin. Radiol.* 18:74-82, 1967.
18. McDonald, P., Hiller, H. G.: Angiography and abdominal tumors in children with particular reference to neuroblastoma and Wilms' tumor. *Clin. Radiol.* 19:1-18, 1968.
19. Nebesar, R. A., Fleischli, D. J., Pollard, J. J., Griscom, N. T.: Arteriography in infants and children with emphasis on Seldinger technique in abdominal disease. *Amer. J. Roent.* 106:81-91, 1969.
20. Nebesar, R. A., Tefft, M., and Filler, R. M.: Correlation of angiography and isotope scanning in abdominal disease of children. *Amer. J. Roent.* 109:323-340, 1970.
21. Palmisano, P. J.: Renal hemartoma (angiomyolipoma): Its angiographic appearance and response to intra-arterial epinephrine. *Radiology* 88:249-252, 1967.
22. Pantoja, E.: Angiography in the liver hemangioma. *Amer. J. Roent.* 104:874-879, 1968.
23. Pollard, J. J., Fleischli, D. J., Nebesar, R. A.: Angiography of hepatic neoplasms. *Radiol. Clin. N. A.* 8:11-41, 1970.
24. Pollard, J. J., Nebesar, R. A., Mattoso, L. F.: Angiographic diagnosis of benign diseases of the liver. *Radiology* 86:276-283, 1966.
25. Poole, C. A., Viamonte, M., Jr.: Unusual renal masses in the pediatric age group. *Amer. J. Roent.* 109:368-379, 1967.
26. Tucker, A. F.: The roentgen diagnosis of abdominal masses in children: Intravenous urography vs. inferior vena cavography. *Amer. J. Roent.* 95:76-90, 1965.
27. Watson, R. C., Baltaxe, H. A.: The angiographic appearance of primary and secondary tumors of the liver. *Radiology* 101:539-548, 1971.
28. Yu, C.: Primary carcinoma of the liver (hepatoma): Its diagnosis by selective celiac arteriography. *Amer. J. Roent.* 99:142-149, 1967.

Nuclear Medicine Imaging Techniques in Childhood Malignancy

August Miale, Jr., M.D.

Radionuclide imaging has been used as a diagnostic tool in adult cancers for many years.[1-5] Only recently, the potential for this diagnostic modality has been realized in children. In the past there was a natural reluctance to administer radionuclides to children because of the possibility of radiation effects. However, advances in instrumentation design and development of short half-life radionuclides have reduced drastically the radiation exposure from these procedures to levels below that obtained with most conventional x-ray examinations.[6] The Anger scintillation camera used in combination with technetium-99m compounds is largely responsible for this change.

The principal use of imaging techniques in cancer patients involves detection of primary or metastatic malignancy either as an initial approach to the patient with suspected but unconfirmed disease or to the patient with known malignancy in whom the question of metastatic involvement must be dealt with. As yet, relatively little progress has been made in cancer detection with radionuclides in patients where cancer is suspected but is only one of several possibilities. This is partially understandable because of the past fears of radiation exposure, which limited development of screening type procedures, and because the vast majority of children with cancer have relatively advanced disease when first seen by a physician. The detection of early disease is extremely difficult because the index of suspicion is low in children until there is a gross manifestation such as overt neurologic deficit, hemorrhage, or evident mass.

Recent trials with radionuclide tracer agents, such as gallium-67 citrate, indium-111 chloride, or iodine-125 iodo quinoline strongly suggest that the quest for a cancer specific localizing agent is rational and may be realized in the next few years.[7] Such agents may become more widely used as a screening approach in children who exhibit even a small degree of deviation from the well-established patterns of nonneoplastic childhood disease. Given the premise that early detection is essential for optimal opportunity for cure, then methods of this type should contribute greatly toward this goal.

August Miale, Jr., M.D., *Associate Professor of Radiology, University of Miami School of Medicine; Chief, Nuclear Medicine Service, Jackson Memorial Hospital, Miami, Fla.*

Unfortunately, the children with cancer encountered in most institutions have relatively advanced disease when the diagnosis is confirmed. The management of these children is difficult, challenging, and success is often related to a total assessment of the patient in terms of the location and extent of the primary and the degree and location of metastasis. Since all forms of cancer therapy depend upon accurate knowledge of the extent of the neoplasm, all the available techniques must be applied as indicated. Serum biochemistry, hematologic, biopsy, and radiographic methods are the current mainstays, but none of these methods suffice for all areas and organs of the body and often fail to delineate sites of cancer or degree of organ involvement.

Cumulative successful experience with radionuclide imaging methods thus far justifies their use for evaluation of all children with known cancer; they are harmless and have shown a remarkable safety record with no mortality or morbidity attributable to the radionuclides. For all practical purposes, there are no contraindications to these techniques.

The remainder of this paper will be devoted to the specific methods which have thus far proven most valuable in contributing to the management of childhood cancer. At this writing, there is only one tracer compound, iodine-125 iodo-quinoline, which is relatively specific for a particular cancer, namely, melanoma. The presence of cancer in various organs causes changes in organ anatomy or local physiologic mechanisms which permit a tracer to concentrate in the abnormal zone or the tracer may be prevented from entering an area involved with disease where it would ordinarily be expected to go. Since various tracers and compounds localize by different mechanisms, some knowledge of the problem in a given patient is needed so as to direct the diagnostic approach most effectively.

Indications

The most common solid malignant tumors of childhood involve liver, brain, kidney, bone, and lymph nodes, and virtually any patient with a known malignancy may develop extension of disease in one or another of these sites at some point in the course of the disease. Assessment of the integrity of these structures can be done by selecting the appropriate imaging techniques. Whenever there is suspicion of primary or secondary involvement of other structures, such as lung, spleen, or thyroid, then appropriate techniques are available for these areas as well.

Pre-Operative

Imaging of various organs prior to surgery is useful to establish a baseline. This is especially valuable in cases likely to involve the liver.[8] The thyroid must be imaged pre-operatively for comparison with postoperative scan in order to determine accurately the amount of residual tissue if a total thyroidectomy is attempted. A patient with osteosarcoma should have a total bone survey with a radionuclide to determine the extent of the primary lesion and the presence of occult metastases. Radiography of bone alone is notoriously insensitive and inaccurate in evaluation of bone metastasis. Recent progress in staging Hodgkin's disease suggests that detection of diseased abdominal mediastinal and supraclavicular nodes can be accomplished accurately with gallium-67 or indium-111 total body scanning. Bone marrow imaging is also helpful in Hodgkin's disease to localize zones of tumor involvement or so-called "skip" areas.[9]

Pre-Radiation Therapy

Some patients will be treated with this modality postoperatively and some directly without surgery. The considerations listed above apply in a similar way. Liver imaging is a simple way to determine the exact zone of radiation effect in the liver. Any approach to local treatment of tumor in bone or bone marrow is enhanced by knowledge of the true extent of disease.[10,11]

Pre-Chemotherapy

As a rule, this form of therapy is likely to be chosen in association or in sequence with the previous methods wherever widespread or systemic disease is present. If chemotherapy is used as the initial and sole form of treatment, the objective indications of response are highly desirable and may be obtained with the appropriate imaging technique.

Follow-up after Treatment

Objective means to assess improvement or regression of disease are limited but considerable information may be obtained by currently available imaging methods. Certain changes cannot be followed easily, for example, regression or widespread hepatic metastases or improvement of leukemic brain involvement.[12-14]

Instrumentation

The most ideal instrument for radionuclide imaging in children is the Anger scintillation camera. The design and utilization of this unique device is extensively described elsewhere.[15] The main advantages of this device over the rectilinear type of scanner are speed, convenience, versatility, and overall superiority of images. Large areas of the body can be surveyed with the camera, especially in small children and infants.

Methods and Radiopharmaceuticals

Brain

Tumors of primary or secondary origin disturb the blood brain barrier and allow certain radiotracers to concentrate in brain to a degree which permits highly accurate localization. The most widely used tracer today is technetium-99m in the form of sodium pertechnetate. Lesions of the posterior fossa and extension of suprasellar lesions, metastasis, and characterization of leukemic infiltration or meningeal seeding all can be detected and characterized.

Liver and Spleen

The reticuloendothelial tissue of liver (Kupfer cells) avidly concentrates colloidal particles tagged with a variety of radiotracers. The most widely used is technetium-99m, tagged sulfur colloid. The homogeneity or integrity of distribution is observed along with liver size and shape. The abnormalities are not specific for tumor but in children with known or suspected cancer, certain patterns are virtually pathognomonic of liver metastasis. The same tracer concentrates in the spleen to a similar degree. Consequently, a tumor of spleen or displacement due to abdominal tumor are readily detected.

Lung

The capillary perfusion bed of the lung will trap macroaggregates of albumin $(10-90\mu)$ labeled with several agents, most popularly technetium-99m or iodine-131. These particles are injected intravenously. Since none of these particles enter the arterial circulation, all can be expected to reside in a pattern indicative of the pulmonary capillary bed. Any which escape to extrapulmonary sites do so because of shunts in the lung or right-to-left intracardiac shunts. Lack of characteristic pattern is always indicative of lung disease. In cancer patients, this most often occurs because of mediastinal node involvement resulting in airway or direct vascular occlusion.

Bone

Certain elements and compounds simulate the metabolic pathways of calcium to a remarkable degree, such that the increased turnover of calcium caused by local tumor in bone is reflected by increased concentration of agents, such as strontium-87m, fluorine-18, and technetium-99m labeled polyphosphates complex. Survey of areas of bone pain reveals positive evidence of metastasis long before x-rays of the same area show abnormalities. Baseline studies in asymptomatic patients also occasionally reveal unsuspected positive sites. The sensitivity and accuracy of bone scanning appear to be substantially superior to routine total body bone survey with x-rays.[4]

Thyroid

The avid concentration of iodine-131 in normal thyroid follows the well-known metabolic pathway of iodine. Less well known is the fact that radioiodine will also concentrate in metastatic thyroid carcinoma provided that most of the normal thyroid is removed at the time of the original surgery. There is no rational basis for partial or subtotal thyroidectomy in children. A total thyroidectomy (with isolation and careful preservation of the parathyroids) results in high endogenous TSH levels and subsequent uptake of radioiodine in the metastatic lesions. Only the highly undifferentiated tumor will not concentrate radioiodine but most if not all of the better differentiated adenocarcinomas in children contain follicular elements which are the basis for radioiodine trapping. Metastatic lesions in remote neck sites, mediastinum, lung and bone are all readily identified with appropriate radioiodine imaging.

Lymph Nodes and Extraorgan Soft Tissue Sites

Localization of malignant tumor in node-bearing areas has been accomplished by new radiotracers which have a propensity to concentrate in the lysozomal fraction of tumor cells. Most significant results have been obtained in patients with lymphoma in whom the presence of tumor in abdominal or thoracic nodes has been established by scanning of either gallium-67 citrate or indium-111 chloride. Future developments along these lines appear to be most promising. For example, the entire evaluation and staging of Hodgkin's disease may be possible with organ imaging techniques alone in association with tissue biopsy identification.

Urinary Tract

Scanning and functional assessment of the kidneys are readily accomplished in children with radiotracers. However, except for Wilm's tumor and rare teratomas, renal imaging has not been frequently employed. Whenever the possibility of a renal tumor exists, screening with scanning methods is indicated because relatively small lesions can be detected, especially when scans are performed with agents such as technetium DTPA and iodine-131 labeled orthoiodohippurate. Following radiation or chemotherapy, questions of secondary effects on the kidney which arise can be dealt with by radiotracer methods.[16]

Bone Marrow

The bone marrow reticuloendothelial (RE) system has the property of trapping a small percentage of intravenously injected radiocolloid. The same material used for liver and spleen scans, namely, technetium-99m sulfur colloid, can be used for revealing the destruction of RE activity in marrow. The RE destruction reflects but is not identified with active hematopoetic tissue destruction. The destruction in normal children is characteristic and any alterations caused by invasion of marrow with tumor are readily discerned. This type of observation has been most helpful in evaluating and staging lymphoma.[9]

Summary

Advances in cancer detection have been made by selected applications of radionuclide organ imaging methods. While the role of these techniques in childhood cancer has only recently been expanded, refinement in instrumentation and tracer compounds show promise of stimulating even more widespread utilization. Because of the insidious nature of neoplasms in children, efforts toward earlier recognition of the disease must be regarded as high priority. The currently available methods as reviewed above can be applied to virtually any child with any known cancer provided the clinical inquiry is properly directed. The challenge for the future lies in establishing acceptable screening methods for detection of the earliest possible manifestation of malignant disease.

References

1. Poulose, K. P., Reba, R. C., Deland, F. H., and Wagner, H. N.: Role of liver scanning in preoperative evaluation of patients with cancer. *Brit. M. J.* 4:585-587, 1969.
2. Ferrante, W. A. and Maxfeld, W. S.: Comparison of diagnostic accuracy of liver scans, liver function tests, and liver biopsies. *South. M. J.* 61:1255-1263, 1968.
3. Johnson, P. C. and Beierwaltes, W. H.: Reliability of scintiscanning nodular goiters judging presence or absence of carcinoma. *J. Clin. Endocr.* 15:865, 1955.
4. Charkes, N. D. and Sklaroff, D. M.: The radioactive strontium photoscan as a diagnostic aid in primary and metastatic cancer in bone. *Radiol. Clin. N. Amer.* 3:499, 1965.
5. Ferrier, F. L., Hatcher, C. R., Achord, J. L., and Abbott, O. A.: Value of liver scanning for detection of metastatic cancer. *Amer. Surgeon* 35:112-120, 1969.
6. Tefft, M.: More common radionuclide examinations in children: Indications for use with a discussion of radiation dose received. *Pediatrics* 48:802, 814, November 1971.
7. Laughammer, H. et al.: ^{67}Ga for tumor scanning. *J. Nuc. Med.* 13:25-30, 1972.
8. Nebesar, R. A., Tefft, M. and Filler, R. M.: Correlation of Angiography and Isotope Scanning in Abdominal Diseases of Children. *Amer. J. Roentgen.* 109:323-340, 1970.
9. Kniseley, R. M., Andrews, G. A., Edwards, C. L., and Hayes, R. L.: Bone-marrow and skeletal scanning. *Radiol. Clin. N. Amer.* 7:265, 1969.
10. Samuels, L. D., Grosfeld, J. L., Kartha, M.: Liver scans after primary treatment of tumors in children. *Surg. Gynec. Obst.* 131:958-964, 1970.
11. Nikaidoh, H., Boggs, J. and Swenson, O.: Liver tumors in infants and children: Clinical and pathologic analysis of 22 cases. *Arch. Surg.* 101:245-257, 1970.
12. David, R. M., Beiler, D., Hood, H. and Morrison, S. S.: Scintillation brain scanning in children. *Amer. J. Dis. Child.* 112:197, 1966.
13. Lorentz, W. B., Simon, J. L. and Benua, R. S.: Brain scanning in children. *JAMA* 201:5, 1967.
14. Mealey, J. Jr.: Brain scanning in childhood. *J. Pediat.*, 69:399, 1966.
15. Gottschalk, A.: Radioisotope scintiphotography with technetium-99m and the gamma scintillation camera, *Amer. J. Roentgen.* 97:860, 1966.
16. Mitus, A., Tefft, M. and Fellers, F. X.: Long-term follow-up of renal functions of 108 children who underwent nephrectomy for malignant disease. *Pediatrics* 44:912-921, 1969.

Diagnosis and Treatment of Childhood Cancer

A Statewide Attack

James L. Talbert, M.D.

Twenty years ago infections far exceeded cancer as a major health hazard. Control and prevention of diseases such as poliomyelitis, diphtheria, pertussis, tetanus and measles now bring cancer to the forefront as a significant medical childhood problem. In fact, today, cancer is surpassed only by accidents as the leading cause of death in children between the ages of one and 14 years in the United States.

While the incidence of childhood cancer has increased somewhat, fortunately it has been matched by major breakthroughs in diagnosis and treatment. It is now possible to cure malignancies in children; malignancies which until recently were considered hopeless.

The rapid changes that are occurring in the field of childhood cancer treatment, however, pose a unique challenge for the practicing physician. First, he has little opportunity to maintain his competence in pediatric cancer care because the overall incidence of neoplasms in this age group is small. Second, the management of cancer in children is fundamentally different from that encountered in later life. In adults, for example, cancer of the lung, stomach, breast, reproductive organs and blood, predominate. Below the age of 15, however, the blood and blood forming organs, bone, kidney, central nervous system, adrenal medulla and eye are the usual sites of involvement. Even cancer of the same organ system may differ in the two age categories. Acute leukemia, for instance, is primarily of the lymphoblastic variety in children, and responds favorably to treatment in more than 90% of patients; in older individuals acute leukemia is usually myelogenous in origin and is more refractory to therapy. Because of these basic age dependent differences in the biology of malignant disease, specialized knowledge is required if children with cancer are to be afforded optimum medical management.

James L. Talbert, M.D., *Professor of Surgery and Chief of Pediatric Surgery, University of Florida College of Medicine, Gainesville, and Coordinator of Florida Regional Medical Program's Children's Cancer Project.*

Reprinted by permission of the *Florida Medical Association,* November 1971 issue.

Children's Cancer Program

As recently as two years ago, few tumor centers in the southeastern United States were staffed with the diversified specialists required for comprehensive care of children with cancer. Since childhood malignancies may involve many different organ systems, the talents of specialists in pediatric surgery, radiotherapy, diagnostic radiology, hematology and oncology, pathology, psychiatry, endocrinology, immunology, and the surgical subspecialties must be available to cope with the complex and diversified problems which may be presented. Only two referral centers in Florida, 350 miles apart at Gainesville and Miami, provided this spectrum of care. Consequently, many of the pediatric cancer patient visits to these clinics each year necessitated travels over long distances. For the children who were ill for long periods, travel four to six hours or more on repeated occasions required unnecessary discomfort and hazard.

Because of these problems of transportation and communication, and because of the need to relate the care of childhood cancer more closely to the practicing physician, the divisions of pediatric surgery, hematology and oncology of the University of Florida College of Medicine initiated organization of a statewide children's cancer program. This proposal received enthusiastic support from the University of Miami School of Medicine and the University of South Florida College of Medicine and from practicing physicians throughout the state. With the interest and participation of these groups, the concept of a statewide program rapidly evolved.

The goals formulated by this group included:

1. Development of a comprehensive statewide Children's Cancer Program utilizing a coordinated network of specialized community units in all major population centers of Florida to work in close liaison with the University of Florida College of Medicine, University of Miami School of Medicine, State Tumor Registry, and University of South Florida College of Medicine in Tampa.

2. Provision of an efficient mechanism for identification and follow-up of children with cancer.

3. Dissemination of information on recent developments in cancer surgery, radiotherapy, and chemotherapy through a planned program in continuing education for community physicians.

4. Organization of a library of pertinent pathological material, x-rays and clinical data on all patients. This compendium of information provides a perpetual source of teaching material and facilitates long-term assessment of treatment regimens.

5. Establishment of an advanced training program in oncology for the development of clinical specialists in the areas of cancer surgery, radiotherapy, chemotherapy, and allied fields.

6. Assurance of adequate attention to the social and economic needs of the affected children and parents and their families through the development of statewide nursing and social service programs devoted exclusively to this problem.

7. Assurance that the most recent advances in basic research related to cancer can be readily available for management of the pediatric tumor patient.

This plan of attack on the problem of childhood tumors was presented to the cancer task force of the Florida Regional Medical Program. Approval and funding was subsequently provided by that organization.

With the cooperation and counsel of Dr. Granville Larimore, State Director of the Florida Regional Medical Program, and Dr. Gordon Engerbretson, Associate State Director, the project was initiated in the summer of 1970. By March 1, 1971 cooperative childhood cancer units were established at Variety Children's Hospital in Miami, University of Miami School of Medicine, Tampa General Hospital (in liaison with the University of South Florida College of Medicine), University of Florida College of Medicine in Gainesville, and Hope Haven Children's Hospital in Jacksonville. Liaison was also established with the Pediatric Clinic of the Pensacola Educational Program, and planning was initiated for development of an additional children's cancer unit in that community. The Pensacola program is scheduled to be activated within the coming year.

Pediatric Tumor Clinics

The staff of each cooperating clinic includes participation by a pediatric hematologist/oncologist, surgeon, radiologist, and radiotherapist. In addition, a variety of pediatric and surgical specialists attend the clinic sessions and participate in patient management.

The five tumor clinics have provided a central consultation service for review of individual patient treatment and for telephone consultation by the community physicians. In addition, literature has been forwarded to physicians regarding individual cases when requested. Tampa and Jacksonville clinics also have inaugurated monthly seminars devoted to specific aspects of children's cancer care; these have been widely attended by community physicians.

The University centers at Miami and Gainesville also have encouraged community physicians from other localities to visit and participate in pediatric tumor clinic sessions in order to expand their knowledge in children's cancer management. In reality, therefore, these physicians are increasing their experience and providing an extension of the University units into their own localities.

In the first six months,* a total of 112 new patients and 1,263 return patient visits were monitored throughout the statewide network of children's cancer clinics. Continuing closed sheets on patient progress are not only maintained by the individual units in the program but through a cooperative liaison which has been established with the State Division of Health, abstracts on all patients are forwarded to the State Central Tumor Registry. Through this system of mutual cooperation, it is anticipated that an accurate evaluation of the incidence of childhood cancer and results of treatment can be provided on a statewide basis.

Childhood Cancer Seminar

In addition to a variety of educational activities which have been inaugurated by the program, both at the local community level and throughout the state, an annual statewide seminar on the problems of childhood cancer is planned. The first such symposium on Pediatric Clinical Oncology will be held at the Miami Sheraton Four Ambassadors Hotel on December 10 and 11, 1971 under sponsorship of the Florida Regional Medical Program's Children's Cancer Project, University of Miami School of Medicine, Division of Radiation Therapy of Cedars of Lebanon Hospital, Department of Therapeutic Radiology in Miami, and the American Cancer Society. Information regarding this symposium may be obtained by writing the central office of the FRMP Children's Cancer Program in Gainesville.

Summary

Cancer in children has assumed increased significance in recent years and represents a major health hazard for this age group. Concomitantly, tremendous strides in diagnosis and treatment have been achieved, and a goal of the FRMP Children's Cancer Project is to provide each child affected by cancer in the state of Florida the latest expertise in the field. No longer is childhood cancer a hopeless condition, but one which, more often than not, poses an excellent prospect of cure.

Information regarding the Florida Regional Medical Program's Children's Cancer Project may be obtained by writing or contacting the following units:

Dr. James L. Talbert, coordinator; or Mr. Joseph C. Price, administrator. Phone: (904) 392-3711, Division of Pediatric Surgery, University of Florida, Box 736 MSB, Gainesville, Florida 32601.

Dr. Kjell Koch, Phone: (305) 371-9611, Division of Pediatrics, University of Miami, Jackson Memorial Hospital, Miami, Florida 33124.

Dr. Albert H. Wilkinson Jr. Phone: (904) 396-2048, Hope Haven Children's Hospital, 5700 Atlantic Blvd., Jacksonville, Florida 32207.

Dr. M. G. Rajurkar. Phone: (305) 666-6511, Department of Pediatrics, Variety Children's Hospital, 6125 S.W. 31st St., Miami, Florida 33155.

Dr. Sorrell L. Wolfson. Phone: (813) 253-0827, 1 Davis Blvd., Davis Islands, Tampa, Florida 33606.

---

*March 1 to August 1, 1971

Staging and Treatment of Neuroblastomas

Audrey E. Evans, M.D.

In considering the staging of tumors one might ask, "What is the value of staging or grouping patients at the time they are first diagnosed?" In answer: It does serve as a real aid to prognosis, it helps to decide the type and amount of treatment and it helps to compare different results with differing regimens. It is always difficult to evaluate the results of someone who says, "This is what I do with my patients and every one of them lives," if at the same time you can't decide what types of patients he is treating. There have been several previously proposed stagings for children with neuroblastoma.[1,2] With advantages and disadvantages in each. By means of 100 patients from two Childrens Cancer Study Group A protocols, I tried to determine their disease pattern and how the stage of disease at diagnosis had affected their prognosis.[3] It seemed clear that a tumor that can be removed completely should be called Stage I and Stage IV designate widespread metastatic disease. We then wondered if there was any advantage in subdividing the localized or regional disease and it appeared that there was a difference depending upon whether or not a tumor crossed the midline. Disease in the abdomen and thorax or involving more than one body cavity affected the prognosis less than bilateral disease.

In the end it appeared that the children who had disease crossing the midline did not do as well as those with unilateral disease even though such tumors were large. We also found that there were some children with metastatic disease who did remarkably well, these were children who had disease in either liver or in the skin, without bone involvement. Such children in Stage IVs and as well as children in Stage I. Table 1 gives the criteria for staging that was devised.

Once the staging was devised, we then studied how well it predicted prognosis. Since age is also an important aspect in the prognosis the patients were also divided according to age. Table 2 gives the results of this analysis. It can be seen from this table that both age and stage of disease at diagnosis do affect survival. A statistical analysis of these 100 patients and a similar group seen at the Children's Hospital of Philadelphia showed that age and stage are

Audrey E. Evans, M.D., *Associate Professor of Pediatrics, University of Pennsylvania; Director, Department of Oncology, The Children's Hospital of Philadelphia, Pa.*

independant variables and both significantly affect the prognosis.[4] Bieslow and McCann's report contains a formula and survival curve which are useful in calculating the chances of survival from the age and stage at diagnosis.

Unfortunately the treatment for neuroblastoma is not nearly as effective as that for Wilms' tumors. The following two points of view express the conventional treatment for neuroblastoma and a more unorthodox viewpoint which is my own. Conventionally, the tumor should be removed, if there is any residual tumor, postoperative irradiation is given to the tumor bed and most people add chemotherapy, certainly, to the 60% of patients who have metastatic disease at diagnosis. This is a particularly sensitive tumor but, unfortunately, chemotherapy does not apparently make a great difference to the median survival time or rate. However, it does relieve symptoms. The combination of cyclophosphamide and vincristine is probably the best. Most children will respond to these two agents for varying lengths of time. We currently administer vincristine in two doses a week apart combined with a fairly high dose of oral cytotoxan until there is significant leukopenia. Most children will tolerate 7-10 days of 10 mg/kg of cytoxan by mouth. It should always be given in the morning and the mother advised to give the child enough fluids to insure that he passes his urine before lunch time in order to minimize bladder toxicity. The 7-10 day course, together with the vincristine is repeated monthly so long as the patient continues to respond.

There is some evidence that adriamycin and daunomycin, two closely allied antibiotics, have a therapeutic effect on neuroblastoma. Tan et al. believe that dannomycin is better than adriamycin as for children with neuroblastomas.[5] We were not so impressed with it when we conducted a study in Group A but the children had far advanced disease.[6] In this study there were 30% subjective responses but no good partial or complete objective responses. However even symptomatic responses improve the quality of survival and the addition of chemotherapy does make life easier for these children even if it does not greatly increase the number who survive.

Now to a more unorthodox view of the treatment. The combined treatment of Wilms' tumor has increased the survival from about 40% to 80%. Why then have we not seen a similar improvement in neuroblastoma? Firstly the percentage of neuroblastoma patients who have distant metastases when first seen is 3 times that of patients with Wilms' tumor (60% vs. 20%). Secondly, the metastatic spread is usually to the skeletal system rather than the lungs. In patients with Wilms' tumor, disease spread to bone has a very poor prognosis and treatment is not nearly so effective as it is for pulmonary metastases. Possibly we have to add a third factor: the immune response of the patient. The Hellstroms have shown that several tumor specific antibodies are produced in response to neuroblastoma, some of which destroy tumor cells in culture and some which block that destruction, thereby protecting the tumor.[7] Vigorous chemotherapy particularly with alkylating agents such as cytoxan may depress the production of effective antibodies.

Dr. Koop at the Children's Hospital of Philadelphia has long been an exponent of limited treatment for children with neuroblastoma.[8] He believes that postoperative radiation therapy is not indicated if little residual tumor remains and that chemotherapy has no value in the asymptomatic patient. The results of treatment of children at his institution are equally as good as those where a more vigorous therapeutic approach is employed. Having reviewed the Children's Hospital cases I have been converted to his philosophy and recommend radiotherapy only if there is considerable residual tumor. Other indications for radiotherapy are painful or unsightly masses to provide relief of suffering. Chemotherapy may also have its place in the management of children with gross residual disease, again to reduce the mass of tumor. Theoretically it should be given in short "bursts" in the hope of increasing the therapeutic ratio and decreasing suppression of an immune response. When our knowledge of these complicated immune reactions improves, some aspects of them could possibly be explored to increase a beneficial type of response and decrease any blocking antibodies. Such measures are still in the future but hopefully not the too distant future.

References

1. Pinkel, D.: Survival in neuroblastoma. *J. Pediat.* 73:928, 1958.
2. Thurman, W. G. and Donaldson, M. H.: *Neoplasia of Childhood.* Chicago:Year Book Medical Publishers, 1967, p. 176.
3. Evans, A. E., D'Angio, G. J., and Randolph, J.: A proposes staging for children with neuroblastoma. *Cancer* 27:374, 1971.
4. Breslow, N. and McCann, B.: Statistical estimation of prognosis for children with neuroblastoma. *Cancer Research* 31:2098, 1971.
5. Tan, C. et al.: Dannomycin, an antitumor antibiotic in the treatment of neoplastic disease. *Cancer* 20:333, 1967.
6. Samuels, L. D., Newton, W. A. and Heyn, R.: Dannorubicin therapy in advanced neuroblastoma *Cancer* 27:831, 1971.
7. Hellstrom, I., Hellstrom, H. E., Bill, A. H., Pierce, G. E., Yang, J. P. S.: Studies on cellular immunity to human neuroblastoma cells, *Int. J. Cancer* 6:172-188, 1970.
8. Koop, C. E., Kieswetter, W. B., and Horn, R. C.: Neuroblastoma in childhood. *Surgery* 38:272, 1955.

Prognosis of Neuroblastoma

Gordon F. Vawter, M.D.

As you have heard, the prognosis of neuroblastoma remains grim. We* are reviewing some 440 neuroblastomas seen since 1919 in the Children's Hospital Medical Center (CHMC) or at the Children's Cancer Research Foundation (CCRF) in Boston. Among patients referred to CHMC for diagnosis and first treatment, the rate of widespread metastases proven at diagnosis was 60%. But for patients first seen at the CCRF the entering rate of widespread dissemination was 82%. These figures indicate how small the salvageable group of patients is at presentation. Hereinafter survival refers to survival more than two years free of known disease.

Causes of Death in Neuroblastoma

It may be worthwhile to remind ourselves of how patients with neuroblastoma die, concentrating on mechanisms of death without previous therapy, so as to give perspective to the effects of therapy.

Obviously, such patients frequently die of disseminated neoplasia, inanition and anemia, but there are other mechanisms of death which may be dealt with, or at least temporized with. Hemorrhage (frequently internal) is an important lethal event: a significant number of such patients have a platelet-trapping neoplasm and consumption coagulopathy: laboratory recognition and therapy of such states will be discussed later in the program.

Other mass lesions apart from inclosed hemorrhage may be lethal, such as massive hepatic metastasis, but they also respond to therapy, sometimes permanently.

Finally, patients with neuroblastoma die of infection, seemingly just as any child in this susceptible age group may died.

Gordon F. Vawter, M.D., *Clinical Assistant Professor of Pathology, Harvard University, Children's Hospital Medical Center, Boston, Mass.*

*Among those contributing in various ways to this review are Drs. J. G. Chi, Robert Filler, R. E. Gross, Norman Jaffe, Herman Polet, Demetrios Traggis as well as Yvonne M. Bishop, Ph.D.

Prognostic Clues in Neuroblastoma

Obviously, a feasible surgical removal has a good prognosis, somewhat less than 100% survival since cryptic metastases to lymph nodes, bone marrow or other sites may be present.

Regardless of site of origin, diagnosis of neuroblastoma under one year of age is associated with a very favorable prognosis. A curious datum emerged from a recent study of primary posterior superior mediastinal neuroblastoma in relation to age at diagnosis: Survival was 100% when diagnosed under one year of age (even in the presence of bilateral or lymph node disease) and 100% when diagnosed over five years of age, the years of risk lying between one and five years at diagnosis. Following this clue, we searched through the larger experience and found preliminary data suggesting that the clinical evolution of neuro-blastoma first diagnosed over five years of age is slower than for neuroblastoma diagnosed at an earlier age.

Undoubtedly everyone here is aware of the favorable prognosis of neuroblastoma primary at sites other than the upper abdomen: notably for mediastinal, cervical or pelvic (presacral) neuroblastoma. To these three perhaps we can add primary spinal neuroblastoma. The problem prognostically is to be sure that tumors presenting at these sites are solitary and not metastases from an upper abdominal primary or to exclude that another primary neuroblastoma remains undiagnosed.

The reasons for the apparently slightly greater salvage of females than males with neuroblastoma noted in this series remain to be analyzed.

Re-emphasizing what Dr. Audrey Evans has already told you is the dismal prognosis for neuroblastomas with known osseous metastasis, our rate of survival under these circumstances approaches, but does not equal zero, namely 0.4%.

Histopathology as a Prognostic Tool

The experience with mediastinal neuroblastoma prompted an analysis of histomorphology as indicator. When the primary tumor consisted of 30% or more of neurofibrillar matrix, survival was 100% for these tumors regardless of age at diagnosis (Table 1). The problem here is the well-known fact that while the primary tumor may be well-differentiated, concomitant lymph node metastases are often less well-differentiated and at the same time bone marrow metastases are likely to be least well-differentiated, albeit perhaps more susceptible to non-surgical therapeutic attack than the better differentiated primary.

As is common in all childhood tumors, in this study of mediastinal neuroblastomas, the presence of high mitotic rates in neuroblastomas diagnosed under one year of age gives little prognostic information, whereas their presence in tumors over one year of age at diagnosis becomes ominous prognostically (Table 2).

TABLE 1. Mediastinal Neuroblastoma

% Neurofibril	% Survival
0-10	33
11-30	60
30+	100

TABLE 2. Mediastinal Neuroblastoma

	% Survival	
	Present	Absent
Calcification	62	33
Mitoses	40	100
Lymphocytes	75	50

Prognosis with Massive Hepatic Neuroblastoma in Infants

In this series there were 45 patients with upper abdominal neuroblastoma and massive hepatic metastases at diagnosis under two years of age (Table 3). Thirty-two of these 45 were under one year old at diagnosis: 21 or 65% of these 32 survive. Among those one to two years old at diagnosis, the survival rate was only 15%, a figure lower than that just given you by Dr. Evans. The reasons for this difference are unclear. Further analyses of this group of 45 patients suggest that we can only account for a portion of those with fatal outcome by discounting those with known osseous metastases at diagnosis. The youngest patient known to me with radiologically diagnosed osseous metastasis was four months old at the time. However, I have seen bone marrow metastases microscopically in newborn infants.

In this connection, analysis of the interval between diagnosis and subsequent metastasis is of interest. For upper abdominal neuroblastoma the average interval between diagnosis and metastasis is about two months. At the other extreme, for primary pelvic neuroblastoma, a smaller group, the average interval between diagnosis and metastasis is about 15 months or seven times longer. In this latter group, as well as those mentioned above as diagnosed beyond the usual age, we

TABLE 3. Hepatic Neuroblastoma under 2 Years Age (Stage IVa)

	Patients			Osseus Metastasis	
	Total	Survivors	%	At Diagnosis	Survivors
Under 1 yr.	32	21	65	5	2
1-2 yr.	13	2	15	9	0
Total	45	23		14	2

should be careful about applying the generally accepted two year survival after diagnosis as index of the patient's success in dealing with his own tumor.

Staging of Midline Neuroblastomas

Dr. Evans and her colleagues have clearly made a major and provocative contribution to the staging of neuroblastoma. You recall that in this system, midline neuroblastomas are considered as bilateral disease, and of grave prognosis. However, we may wish to revise this estimate somewhat when the results with certain midline neuroblastomas are considered (Table 4).

There were 10 survivors of 16 with primary pelvic neuroblastoma. Of six under one year of age at diagnosis, four survived, three of three survived in the one to two year age group and about 50% of those diagnosed over two years of age survived. Curiously, there was an apparently high proportion of females bearing this tumor.

Let's turn to another midline neuroblastoma, the spinal neuroblastoma. In this series, these are defined as neuroblastomas which, at the time of diagnosis, were treated surgically for spinal mass. Nine out of 24 (or 36%) of such patients survive. Of these nine: five were thoracic, three were lumbar and one was pelvic; four were under one year of age at diagnosis and four had no other paraspinal mass. All, of course, received other therapy including radiation and chemotherapy.

TABLE 4. Midline Neuroblastoma (Stage III)

	Survivors	Total	%
Spinal	9	24	36
Pelvic	10	16	62

What Is, in Fact, a Neuroblastoma?

Ultimately, prognostics in neuroblastoma will improve, I believe, when we are able to distinguish between histologically indistinguishable primitive tumors of neural crest origin: these are all presently called neuroblastoma but probably include tumors arising in dorsal sensory spinal ganglia, sympathetic ganglia, adrenal medulla, chromaffin tissue which accompanies sympathetic ganglia and parasympathetic ganglia among others.

Each one of these tissues undoubtedly has differing potentials and pressures for differentiation.

Adequately proven parasympathetic neuroblastomas are exceedingly rare, but their relatively peripheral origin may aid in complete surgical excision at certain sites. By analogy with the generally benign behavior of chromaffin tumor of adults, we may suspect that chromaffin cell neuroblastomas may have somewhat analogous behavior. Other hypothetical analyses could be offered for the rest of the group of neuroblastomas.

However, to distinguish these differing neoplasms will probably require methods of analysis not yet generally applied, such as biochemical, immunologic or tissue culture parameters.

Pulmonary Metastases in Wilms'

I. G. Williams, M.B., F.R.C.S., F.F.R.

The lungs are the commonest site of metastases in Wilms' tumour and the route is via the blood stream. Both the sarcomatous and epithelial elements are malignant, and embryonic, and rich in blood supply, the blood spaces communicating with the renal veins. In some, the cancer clumps can be seen in the capsular veins and extending into the renal veins as a malignant thrombus. The route of spread is evident microscopically, sometimes macroscopically.

The lesson from this is twofold:

1. Minimal palpation in examination and gentleness in surgery.
2. Dissemination is mechanical and the route must be closed mechanically and urgently with a ligature round the renal veins and nephrectomy.

Having reached the blood stream the malignant emboli settle in the lungs. It may be a single embolus that survives or as is more common multiple — the bilateral cannon ball metastases. If they filter through, they can settle in bone, or metastasise generally. Widespread abdominal liver and pulmonary metastases are due to overwhelming spread by all the classical routes. The importance of the lungs is that for a time, in some, they may be the only site of metastases. As such they could be amenable to treatment. It is, therefore, our duty to try to assess:

1. The full extent of the disease in the patient as he or she presents.
2. To try also in all patients without evident spread at the time they come to us, to determine those conditions where spread may be either (a) unlikely, or (b) likely. (a) Unlikely: in order to minimise our traumatic, toxic or iatrogenic therapies. (b) Likely: here we have to do everything we can, without damage, to cure the child.

The treatment of pulmonary metastases may therefore be classified as (1) Definitive, (2) Prophylactic.

Definitive Pulmonary Metastases

The types of metastases in the lungs from a Wilms' tumour fall into one of three categories:

I. G. Williams, M.B., F.R.C.S., F.F.R., *Consultant Radiotherapist St. Bartholomew's Hospital and the Hospital For Sick Children, Great Ormond Street, London, England.*

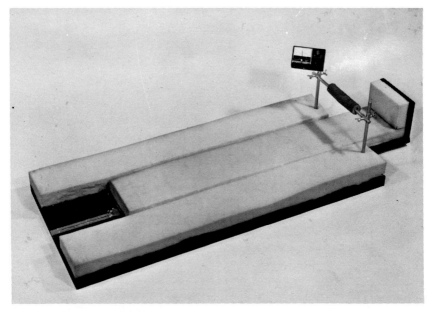

Fig. 1. Board and adapted head rest for anaesthetised children under Cobalt therapy. (Designed by Dr. T. Boulton.)

Widespread bilateral and miliary

This occurs with generalised dissemination throughout the body and there is nothing further we can do about it.

A single solitary embolic deposit

If this can be defined and others excluded, this, if suitable, could be removed surgically.

Bilateral cannonball metastases

Growing experience seems to indicate that for a time at least there are some patients, however widespread in the lungs – the lungs appear to be the only sites. As such the problem then amounts to destruction of these deposits by the agents at our disposal, irradiation and chemotherapy, without damage to the lung.

The patients with pulmonary metastases can be divided into two groups:

A. Those that have pulmonary metastases at the first consultation or presentation, and

B. Those with clear chests at first presentation but who develop metastases later on, in the follow-up period after the primary treatment is completed. It is a study of these which might indicate to us those who are very prone later to develop metastases.

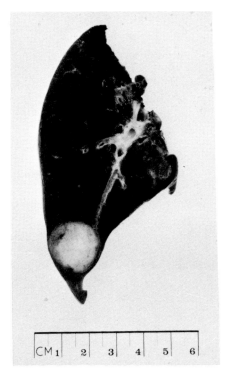

Fig. 2. Single pulmonary metastasis removed by resection.

Our treatment method in these groups has been as follows:

Surgical: Single metastases are removed either by lobectomy or a wedge resection of the affected part of the lung. We have never done a pneumonectomy in a child.

Radiotherapy: Because of the obvious known advantages we use either Cobalt 60 or 4 MeV accelerator megavoltage irradiation. We deliver the tolerance dose of the normal lung and the total dose and overall time will depend upon what we believe this to be. We give 1500 r evenly throughout both lungs in 12 days. It is important to cover the entire lung, the gutters around the diaphragm and the apices and to protect the humeral epiphyses. We give the full fraction on the first day and it is quite astonishing how the children stand up to this. Radiation sickness has not been a serious problem in our experience.

Chemotherapy: We used Actinomycin D (or Vincristine). With such irradiation the dose of Actinomycin D employed has been 60 micrograms/Kg. body weight divided into 4 fractions. In this group it was given at the end of irradiation. The fall in white and platelet count then occurs before we can worry about what is happening.

Personal Series

Between January 1st 1960 and December 31st 1969 we treated 81 children with Wilms' tumours. Thirty-five of these (4.3%) either had or developed pulmonary metastases:

At presentation 13 : 16%

Appeared later 22 : 27%

At Presentation Total 13. 16% of the total.

All these children were over the age of 3 years and apart from one they all had large primary tumours adherent in the renal bed, to bowel or to diaphragm.

Case 1. Male aged 5. Single metastasis treated by surgery.

One days's history of an enlarged abdomen noted by mother. Single metastasis in periphery of right upper lobe. Nephrectomy. Encapsulated tumour. No spread. No infiltration.

No venous involvement.

Two weeks later – wedge resection.

Postoperative irradiation to lungs only. No chemotherapy because of leucopenia (2500 – 3000). Thrombocytopenia 140,000. We treated what we thought was most important. Alive and well and free 4 (4 10/12) years.

Multiple Metastases: 12

1 alive and well 6 years. 11 died. (2 Stage 5 – bilateral. 9 Stage 4). One girl aged 6. Two weeks abdominal pain. Huge left tumour. Multiple bilateral lung metastases. A.C.D. 1450 μg in 5 days. Nephrectomy: Splenectomy: Trans-colectomy. Irradiation – chest 1500 r., renal bed 3500 r. Four weeks later further A.C.D. Alive and well – 6 years.

Metastases Appearing Later

At the first consultation there were 68 patients who had a normal chest X-ray. Tomography had not been done in any of these as a routine, but I believe now should be done as a skeletal survey is done in neuroblastoma.

Metastases appeared in   22 = 33%

Within 3 months in   6

3-9 months in   13 = 19 within 9 months.

Over 1 year – 3. The longest was 43/12. (Aged 10).

Metastasis was a single deposit in 2.

Both treated by surgery – one alive 2 years,

one died 4/12 – generalised disease.

Metastases were multiple in 20 (of the 22 that appeared later)

Surgery

Surgery played a part in the treatment of 3 of these, but in various sequences they also had irradiation and chemotherapy. Surgery was used when we thought

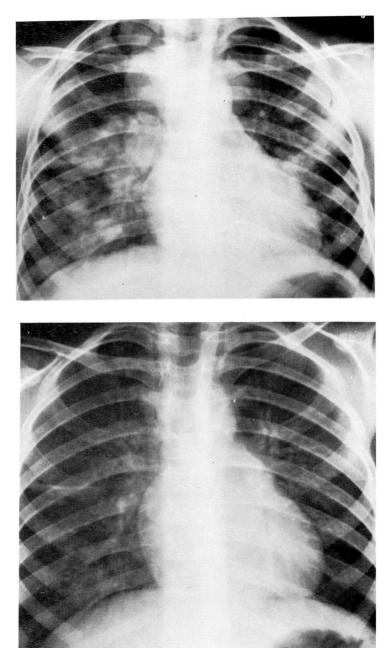

Figs. 3 and 4. Cannonball metastases in both lungs to show the effects of pulmonary irradiation – 1500 r. in 2 weeks.

lung and/or haemopoietic tolerance had been reached – or when a metastasis appeared within irradiated tissue.

Two of these are alive and well and tumour free at 5 years, and one died in the first year.

Appeared later

In 17 patients where the metastases appeared in the follow-up period and were bilateral and multiple only two survive. They are alive, well and tumour free 4 and 2 years after therapy.

Summary of All Cases

Of the 81 children with Wilms' tumours 54% were alive and well at 2 years, and 49% up to 9 years.

Treatment of Pulmonary Metastases

Surgery 6. Alive 4. (5,4,3 and 3 years).

Radiotherapy and Chemotherapy 29. Alive 3 at 6, 4 and 3 years.

Seven children out of 35 i.e. 20% with pulmonary metastases have survived and are alive and well. These statistics include all children with Wilms' tumour in whom radical treatment was given with the aim to cure, albeit ill-judged perhaps in some of the Stage 4 and 5 cases, but at least the attempt was made.

References

Stone, J. and Williams, I. G.: "The treatment of Wilms' tumour with special reference to Actinomycin D. *Clinical Radiology* XX, 1:40-46, 1969.

Central Nervous System Neoplasia in Childhood

Stuart B. Brown, M.D.

Primary tumors of the brain represent the third most common form of childhood neoplasia, exceeded only by the leukemias and the renal-perirenal tumor group. The mortality rate from such nervous system tumors is second only to that seen with the leukemias. Therefore, central nervous system neoplasia in childhood is a relatively common problem whose solution may be difficult due to the anatomic localization, unusual natural history and variable responsiveness of these tumors to therapy.

In the adult, brain tumors are primarily supratentorial in location, whereas in childhood, tumors are more common to the posterior fossa and suprasellar areas. Because of this localization, the symptom complex seen in children with brain tumors tends to be different from that seen in adults, and the therapeutic problems surrounding these tumors are more complicated than that experienced in tumors of cerebral localization. The following discussion will be limited to neoplasms located outside the cerebral hemispheres.

Gliomas make up the largest portion of brain tumors in childhood. These are primarily of low grade, as opposed to a much greater incidence of high grade gliomas, such as glioblastoma multiforme, that are noted in adults. The most common non-cerebral tumor of the glioma series seen in childhood is the cerebellar astrocytoma. This is followed in incidence in the glioma series by medulloblastomas, brain stem gliomas, ependymomas and optic gliomas. The most common nongliomatous tumor in childhood is the craniopharyngioma which is the third or fourth most common brain tumor in the overall group.

These tumors are located in the paraxial and periventricular regions of the brain. Craniopharyngiomas, optic gliomas, gliomas of the hypothalamus, dermoids, and teratomas are all localized about the sella turcica and optic chiasm with a potentiality for encroachment on the anterior part of the third ventricle. Brain stem gliomas, medulloblastomas, cerebellar astrocytomas and fourth ventricular ependymomas encroach upon the aqueduct of sylvius and fourth ventricle again because of their paraxial location.

Stuart B. Brown, M.D., *Assistant Professor of Neurology & Pediatrics University of Miami School of Medicine, Miami, Florida.*

The mid-line localization of these tumors causes symptoms of headache, vomiting, irritability and diplopia. These symptoms are nonspecific, but when combined with signs such as papilledema, abducens nerve palsies, positive MacEwen's sign (crack pot sign) and cranial enlargement they immediately indicate increased intracranial pressure secondary to encroachment on the ventricular system. Therefore, the location of these neoplasms produces a nonspecific symptom complex indicative of raised intracranial pressure. The presence of additional signs and symptoms enables the physician to localize the site of the problem. Visual apparatus abnormalities such as amblyopia, optic atrophy or bitemporal visual field deficits localize the problem to the region of the optic nerves or chiasm. Endocrine problems such as short stature, delayed or precocious puberty suggest localization in the hypothalamic region of the brain. Multiple bilateral cranial nerve palsies, and corticospinal and cerebellar signs in combination indicate an intrinsic brain stem lesion usually originating in the area of the pons. The presence of neck stiffness, head tilt, and suboccipital tenderness suggest a problem in the region of the foramen magnum and cysterna magna.

Ataxia is a very prominent sign in central nervous neoplasms in childhood. Inasmuch as approximately 60% of such tumors are located in the posterior fossa, the presence of ataxia, or unsteadiness of gait, is not an unusual finding, and its presence immediately suggests a cerebellar lesion. It is important to be aware of the fact that this symptom need not arise from the cerebellum per se, but may be seen with lesions of the cerebellar pathways as well. Lesions of the afferent cerebellar pathways in the pons and medulla may give rise to ataxia as may lesions of the cerebellar outflow tract, or lesions in the cerebellar projection areas of the thalamus and frontal lobe. Increased intracranial pressure and cerebellar ataxia, therefore, are seen commonly as the presenting symptoms or major neurological signs in children with neoplasms that abut on the brain stem, diencephalon, or mid-line ventricular areas.

Cerebellar astrocytomas represent the most frequently seen posterior fossa neoplasm. They are seen primarily in the first decade of life with a peak incidence in the second half of this decade. They present with signs of increased intracranial pressure and cerebellar dysfunction. Their rate of growth is generally slow, thus making possible a prolonged duration of symptoms prior to diagnosis. These tumors may be solid, but have a great tendency to become cystic. They are potentially curable surgically if the solid portion of the tumor can be removed. Generally, the surgical cure rate is excellent. Incomplete removal of this tumor is compatible with prolonged survival with radiation therapy being used post-operatively. However, the meaningfulness of radiation therapy in such a slow growing and well differentiated neoplasm is open to question.

Medulloblastomas represent the most malignant and rapidly growing tumor of the central nervous system. This tumor is seen in the first decade with a peak incidence in the first half of the decade. The lesion presents clinically with symptoms of increased intracranial pressure of very recent onset. Complete surgical removal of this tumor appears to be impossible, thus necessitating postoperative irradiation to the entire cranium and spinal axis. The latter therapy is essential, as the tumor has the ability to seed along the cerebrospinal fluid pathways with the tumor cell surviving free in the cerebrospinal fluid. Ultimately, the cells attach to a distant point along the neuraxis and multiply producing symptoms referable to this location. Intrathecal chemotherapy has at times been helpful in treatment of symptoms arising from such seeding. Prognosis is poor with most patients succumbing within two years of the time of diagnosis. However, there are indications that five to ten year survival rates may be attained in 30% to 40% of the patients with a combination of surgery and radiation therapy.

Brain stem gliomas represent an entity easily diagnosed as long as the possibility of the lesion is considered. It is seen primarily in the first decade with a peak incidence of about six or seven years of age. Signs of increased intracranial pressure are rarely present until late in the course of this lesion. Bilateral cranial nerve palsies, primarily of the sixth and seventh cranial nerves, are seen early, and are associated with unilateral or bilateral corticospinal and cerebellar signs. The onset of these symptoms is insidious and the overall growth rate of the tumor is slow. Diagnosis can be made with pneumoencephalography as the increased mass of the pons is manifested by narrowing of the prepontine cistern and posterior displacement of the floor of the fourth ventricle. Because this neoplasm is intrinsic within the brain stem, surgical intervention is impossible. Recent evidence indicates that irradiation therapy is capable of producing improvement in clinical status and prolonging survival to a degree three times greater than in untreated patients. Average survival with radiation therapy has been approximately four years with 18 to 19 year survivals occasionally seen.

Craniopharyngiomas represent the most common nongliomatous neoplasm seen in the central nervous system in childhood. These tumors can be seen at any age with the majority being noted in the first or second decade. The peak incidence appears to be in the middle of the first decade. Symptoms and signs are primarily those of increased intracranial pressure, visual loss, bitemporal visual field deficit, and short stature. Decrease in growth hormone production and thyroid function is not uncommon here. Suprasellar calcification is seen on skull x-ray in pratically all children with this tumor, and x-rays for determination of bone age often reveal delay in skeletal maturation. Treatment of this tumor is somewhat controversial because of the permanence of serious endocrine problems that often arise in the postoperative period. Total surgical removal is advocated by some and subtotal removal and postoperative radiation therapy by others. Inasmuch as these tumors are cystic, a third group advocates surgical biopsy and cyst evacuation followed by radiation therapy. Long term survival has been seen in each of these therapeutic approaches leaving the issue to date unsettled.

Optic gliomas are very slowly progressive tumors situated in the optic nerve unilaterally or bilaterally or in the optic chiasm. They present usually as a unilateral decrease or loss of vision in one eye, and in young children, this may be manifested by a unilateral strabismus due to the amblyopia in that eye. If the lesion is in the intraorbital portion of the nerve, proptosis may be the presenting symptom and sign. If the chiasm is involved, a bitemporal visual field deficit may be noted on examination. These lesions may extend upward into the hypothalamus producing precocious puberty, and they may ultimately produce increased intracranial pressure secondary to further encroachment on the third ventricle. Optic atrophy is common, and this may be unilateral or bilateral. Optic foramen enlargement with decrease in visual acuity and optic atrophy in a child under ten years of age, and especially under five years of age, is suggestive of this entity. Therapy is again controversial. Surgical intervention appears appropriate in gliomas localized to the intraorbital portion of the optic nerve. Those lesions involving the intracranial portion of one optic nerve but clearly separate from the chiasm have been removed surgically at the expense of the optic nerve. Bilateral optic nerve involvement and chiasmatic involvement are not amenable to surgical therapy. Subtotal surgical removal of this tumor, surgical biopsy with postoperative irradiation, or irradiation therapy alone may result in long term survival with stabilization of vision, irrespective of the type of therapy administered. Recent reviews indicate that stabilization of the visual deficit, or even improvement in vision may occur with no treatment at all, suggesting that the natural history of this tumor is the same, with or without any form of therapy. In as much as vision may be worsened by surgical biopsy or irradiation therapy, the best approach to the treatment of optic gliomas may be careful serial observation and examination without initial definitive therapy. If progression ensues, then radiation therapy would appear to be indicated. It is also important to realize that this tumor is seen frequently in neurofibromatosis and may be only the initial manifestation of this neurocutaneous disease.

The chemotherapeutic approach to brain tumors is being utilized in some medical centers with the use of intrathecal agents, isolated vascular perfusion techniques, and direct implantation of chemical or radioactive agents into the tumors. To date, these techniques or agents have not been found to be superior to other forms of therapy.

In summary, cerebral tumors in childhood are a relatively common and serious medical problem. Sixty to seventy percent of these neoplasms lie outside the cerebral hemispheres with the majority located in the posterior fossa. Encroachment on the ventricular pathway because of the paraxial location of these tumors leads to signs and symptoms of increased intracranial pressure. Additional signs and symptoms permit exact localization of the tumor and neuroradiological studies and surgical biopsy allow for determination of tumor type. Therapy is then individualized according to the natural history of the specific tumor and its responsiveness to the various modes of available therapy.

References

1. Matson, D. D.: *Neurosurgery of Infancy and Childhood.* 2nd Ed, Springfield, Ill.:Chas. C Thomas, 1969.
2. Aron, Bernard S : Medulloblastoma in Children. *Amer. J. Dis. Child.* 121:314-317, 1971.
3. Matson, Donald D. and Crigler, J. F.: Management of Craniopharyngioma in Childhood. *J. Neurosurg.* 30:377-390, 1969.
4. Kramer, Simon, Southard, M., and Mansfield, C. M.: Radiotherapy in the Management of Craniopharyngiomas. *Amer. J. Roentgen.* 103:44-52, 1968.
5. Panitch, Hillel S., and Berg, B. O.: Brain Stem Tumors of Childhood and Adolescence. *Amer. J. Dis. Child.* 119:465-472, 1970.
6. Hoyt, William and Baghdassarian, S. A.: Optic Gliomas in Childhood. *Brit. J. Ophth.* 53:793-798, 1969.
7. Glaser, Joel, Hoyt, Wm, and Corbett, J.: Visual Morbidity with Chiasmal Gliomas. *Arch. Ophth.* 85:3-12, 1971.

Rhabdomyosarcoma in Childhood

R. D. T. Jenkin, M.B., F.R.C.P. (C)

Rhabdomyosarcoma is the commonest soft tissue sarcoma of childhood (Table 1). In a series of 101 tissue sarcomas seen at The Princess Margaret Hospital, Toronto, rhabdomyosarcoma accounted for 70 patients, and in a further 13 the histological diagnosis was unspecified sarcoma where the sarcomatous pattern was too poorly differentiated to permit further categorization. These 83 patients were all treated in the same fashion and will be analyzed together.

It is especially difficult to categorize a poorly differentiated sarcoma when the primary site of origin is paraspinal, related to the chest wall, or is in the retroperitoneum (Table 2). The differentiation from Ewing's sarcoma is especially difficult at these sites. Neuroblastoma is now only rarely a cause for difficulty in the differential diagnosis in the paraspinal regions, since the abnormal pattern in the urinary excretion of catecholamines and their metabolites may readily be detected.

The well-known pattern of distribution by site of rhabdomyosarcoma in childhood is shown in Table 3. Tumours arising in the head and neck region and in the pelvis are the two dominant groups in this series. Approximately 30% of our patients are alive with follow-up intervals ranging from 1-13 years.

The prospects for cure in rhabdomyosarcoma have improved in recent years and this may be seen (Fig. 1) when we compare the patients treated from 1958 to 1965, to those treated from 1966 to 1970. In the more recent group 50%, or 13 of 26 patients, are alive at three years, compared to 21% for the earlier years. Whilst these are crude comparisons we could detect no obvious difference in the patients in the two groups. Both groups contained approximately 20% of patients with metastatic disease at diagnosis, both groups contained about the same proportions of patients in whom only a biopsy or partial excision of the tumour had been undertaken and there was no obvious asymmetry in the more favourable sites between the two groups. Patients are referred to The Princess Margaret Hospital for irradiation or chemotherapy so this is a select group of patients which omits both ends of the spectrum. On the one hand patients treated by a complete surgical procedure only, and on the other, patients with

R. D. T. Jenkin, M.B., F.R.C.P. (C) *The Ontario Cancer Institute incorporating The Princess Margaret Hospital, Toronto.*

TABLE 1. Soft Tissue Sarcoma — Age < 16 yrs.
PMH 1958-1970*

Rhabdomyosarcoma Inc. Malig. Mesenchymoma	70
Sarcoma Unspecified	13
Fibrosarcoma	10
Other Specific Sarcoma	8
Total	101

*The distribution of histological type in the soft tissue sarcoma of childhood as seen at The Princess Margaret Hospital, Toronto, a referral centre for the medical management of malignant disease.

TABLE 2. Rhabdomyosarcoma — Age < 16 yrs.
PMH 1958-1970*

	Site	
	Chest Wall Spine Retroperitoneum	Other
Rhabdomyosarcoma Inc. Malig. Mesenchymoma	7	63
Sarcoma Unspecified	8	5

*The variation of the histological diagnosis with the anatomical site of the primary tumour is demonstrated.

TABLE 3. Rhabdomyosarcoma — Age < 16 yrs.*

Primary Site	No. Patients	No. Alive
Head & Neck	31	10
Trunk	15	4
Pelvis & Genitalia	24	6
Limb	12	4
Bile Ducts	1	0
Total	83	24

*Distribution by site of rhabdomyosarcoma and unclassified soft tissue sarcoma. The number of patients diagnosed and the number alive (1.11.71.) is shown for each site.

overwhelming disease which prevented transfer to a specialist hospital, are omitted.

When we compare, for these two time intervals, the survival curve and the curve demonstrating the proportion of patients free of metastatic or recurrent disease, we see (Fig. 2) for 1958-1965 that recurrence happened usually in the first six months and nearly always within the first year. In more recent years (Fig. 3) fewer patients recurred but the time of recurrence was very little changed.

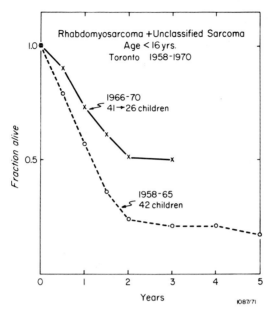

Fig. 1. Crude survival is compared for children diagnosed during the years 1958-1965 and 1966-1970.

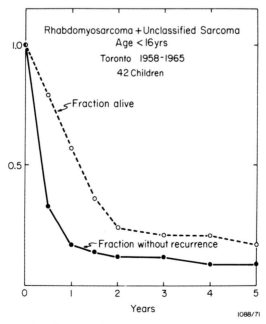

Fig. 2. A comparison of the fraction of children alive with the fraction free of recurrence for those diagnosed in the years 1958-1965.

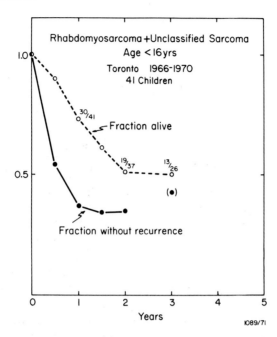

Fig. 3. A comparison of the fraction of children alive with the fraction free of recurrence for those diagnosed in the years 1966-1970.

Treatment Variables

Let us consider now the manner in which these patients were treated and the evolution of our treatment methods during these years. All patients referred to us had undergone a surgical procedure, most often a simple biopsy alone (B), less often a partial removal of the tumour (P), and occasionally a complete surgical removal (C), though in a proportion of these cases there were grounds for supposing that there was microscopic residual disease (MR). All received post-operative irradiation. We asked the question "Did the extent of the surgical procedure influence our cure rate?" In Table 4 the extent of surgery is related to the number of children alive and to the number dead, but separating in the latter group those in whom the primary was controlled until death. (The total of 64 children in this analysis is small because not all our children were followed closely to death and in a proportion the state of the primary site at death was not known.) It can be seen that primary control was more likely if all (C) or most (MR) of the tumour had been removed. Thus, the primary remains controlled or was controlled until death in 11 of 15 children when no more than microscopic residual disease remained following surgery, whereas control was achieved only in 18 of 49 children subjected to biopsy (B) or partial tumour removal (P). The numbers available do not permit an analysis by site in addition,

TABLE 4. Rhabdomyosarcoma — Age < 16 yrs.*

	Alive	Dead	
Extent of Surgery	Primary Controlled	Primary Controlled	Primary Recurrent
B	6	9	25
P	3	0	6
MR	4	3	3
C	3	1	1
	26 - 120 mos.	3 - 56 mos.	

*The relationship between extent of surgery and control at the primary site is demonstrated (see text).

although it is obvious that it is the worst tumours in the least accessible sites that discourage more than a biopsy. These results also make it quite clear that post-operative irradiation offers some chance of cure even when the surgical procedure is limited to biopsy.

The manner of irradiation changed during the course of this study. In the early years modest volume modest dose techniques were employed and in later years generous volume high dose techniques. These two factors have been analyzed separately. Comparison of the relative volume irradiated with success or failure in control of the primary tumour demonstrated a differing pattern. Relatively large volumes of irradiation were associated with success and small volumes with failure (Table 5).

TABLE 5. Rhabdomyosarcoma — Age < 16 yrs.*

	Relative Volume Irradiated		
Primary Tumour Status	Large %	Medium %	Small %
Controlled (28 pts.)	64	29	7
Recurrent (33 pts.)	46	21	33

*Comparison of the relative volume irradiated with success or failure in control of the primary tumour.

Soft tissue sarcomas are often much more extensive than is apparent by inspection and palpation and therefore it is important to undertake a complete investigation of every patient to determine the anatomical extent of their disease. It is important to err on the side of treating too large a volume rather than too small, for if any part of a tumour is untreated the chance of survival is zero.

The dose/time relationships for irradiation of primary sites in the head, neck and limbs is shown (Fig. 4). In 10 of 13 patients below the line, the primary

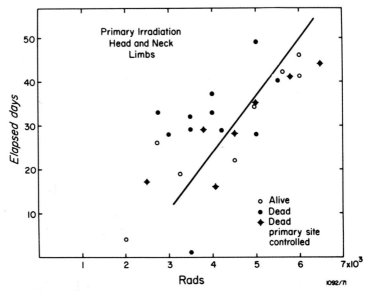

Fig. 4. Time/Dose relationships for primary irradiation. Head, neck and limb tumours.

tumour was controlled either to the present time or to the death of the patient, whereas primary control was obtained only in 5 of 13 patients at the lower doses represented above the line. The data for primary tumours of the orbit is shown separately (Fig. 5). Using an identical line of demarcation seven of ten patients given the higher doses represented beneath the line obtained primary tumour control. Lower doses of irradiation were used for tumours arising in the pelvis and trunk (Fig. 6). Tumour control was obtained in 5 of 22 patients given the lower doses represented above the line. Lower doses were used in these patients because of the large volume of tissue being irradiated and oftentimes because it was not anticipated that the treatment would have any but a palliative function.

These dose time data make it clear that for a reasonable chance of permanent control in rhabdomyosarcoma a high dose, for example not less than 5,000 rads in five weeks, is necessary.

Appropriate surgery and irradiation without chemotherapy offers only a fair chance of cure in rhabdomyosarcoma. In this series, of our 24 surviving patients, 22 are trouble free and have a good chance of cure. Of these only four received chemotherapy at any stage in their disease, so that the survival curves presented can fairly be said to be those obtainable with surgery and irradiation alone with respect to the final cure rate. The manner in which irradiation is used for a solitary recurrence is also very important. For of our 22 long term survivors, five were controlled after recurrence: one after recurrence at the primary site, two after the development of regional lymph nodes, one after development of pulmonary metastasis, and one after development of a secondary lesion in a rib.

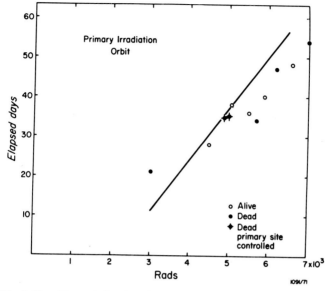

Fig. 5. Time/Dose relationships for primary irradiation. Orbital tumours.

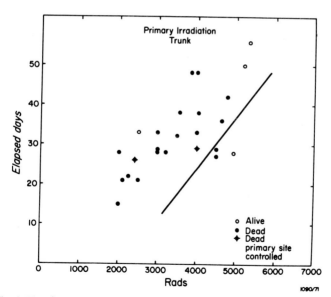

Fig. 6. Time/Dose relationships for primary irradiation. Trunk including pelvis.

Over the years of this study, chemotherapy has become increasingly important. It has been known now for several years that Actinomycin D, Vincristine and Cyclophosphamide each have a good chance of producing an objective response in the metastatic phase of this disease. For the greater part of the time covered by this study we did not give chemotherapy electively, but reserved it for treatment of recurrence. Good palliation and useful prolongation of life is obtained with these agents. Thus of 56 patients dying of metastatic rhabdomyosarcoma, 47 received chemotherapy and their survival ranged from one to 40 months from the time of their first recurrence, with an average survival of ten months, and a median of nine months. In comparison, nine patients who received no chemotherapy survived one to five months, with an average of three months from the time of the first recurrence.

Whilst excellent remissions may be obtained with these agents late in the disease, and used sequentially, cures are probably not obtained. However evidence is building that the elective use of these agents in the most favourable group of patients, where the surgical removal has been grossly complete and post-operative irradiation given, may appreciably increase the survival rate.

Experience with elective chemotherapy in this series is limited to 19 patients. Five of these patients remain alive although two have required treatment for recurrence. These patients are a selected unfavourable group in that the most favourable sites in our experience, the orbit and paratesticular structures, were not included in the electively treated group.

Malignant Bone Tumours of Childhood

R. D. T. Jenkin, M.B., F.R.C.P.(C)

Osteosarcoma

Sixty-two patients with osteosarcoma were seen at The Princess Margaret Hospital, Toronto, from 1958-1970. When we examine the age-incidence of this tumour (Fig. 1) we see that 42 of these patients were less than 30 years old, with a peak incidence at 10-14 years. It is the management of this group of patients that I shall consider. In 30 of these 42 patients the primary site was in the lower limb distal to the mid-femur (Fig. 2). In comparison only one of 20 tumours in older patients occurred in this part of the leg. Thus in the younger group, in three of every four patients, we are concerned with management of a distal lower limb tumour.

Thirty-eight of the patients have been followed for more than six months from diagnosis. The crude survival curve and the curve showing the proportion of patients without clinically demonstrable metastatic disease is given (Fig. 3). It is clear that metastases appear early, most often at the time of diagnosis or within six months. Only two patients remained free of metastatic disease and are probably cured. It is apparent that we have no good treatment method.

It is generally held that the cure rate in osteosarcoma is the same whether treatment is by immediate radical surgery or by radical irradiation followed by selective radical surgery: at six months, for the group of patients in whom the primary is controlled and who remain free of metastatic disease, or at an earlier time if there is primary recurrence and no metastatic disease. We have most often followed this second course on the premise that radical irradiation will provide good local palliation and thus avoid unnecessary amputations for the majority who will succumb to pulmonary metastases during the first year. We have examined our data to see whether this premise is sound.

Of the 42 patients, ten were treated by immediate surgery with one apparent cure; 29 were treated by radical irradiation and selective amputation also with one cure, and three with metastases at diagnosis were treated palliatively.

R. D. T. Jenkin, M.B., F.R.C.P.(C), *The Ontario Cancer Institute, The Princess Margaret Hospital, Toronto, Canada.*

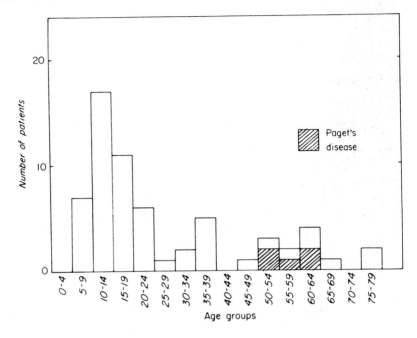

Fig. 1. Osteosarcoma. Age Incidence.

In the group of patients eligible for the combined treatment, the volume of tissue irradiated included the whole tumour with a generous margin, particularly along the proximal shaft of a long bone, though only occasionally was the whole bone irradiated. A Cobalt unit was utilized in every case.

The response of the primary tumour was classified as complete when there were no residual symptoms and no palpable tumour following irradiation; as partial when there was only a decrease in symptoms and/or tumour size, and as no response when neither symptoms nor size improved.

Data was adequate to assess the response in 27 patients. The response to irradiation was poor (Table 1). A complete response was seen in three, a partial response in 17, and no response in seven. Moreover, the primary tumour recurred in all 27 patients. This was grossly evident in a mean time of 5.5 months for those with a partial response, and in four months for the three patients with a complete response. A distinction between partial response and complete response was therefore not of value. The dose used (Fig. 4) ranged from 4,500 rads in three weeks to 7,000 rads in seven weeks, close to tissue tolerance for the chosen time interval. Eight patients with distal limb tumours were treated under hypoxic conditions. All showed a partial tumour response which was not superior to the response in the conventionally irradiated patients. A further increase in dose would not be practical.

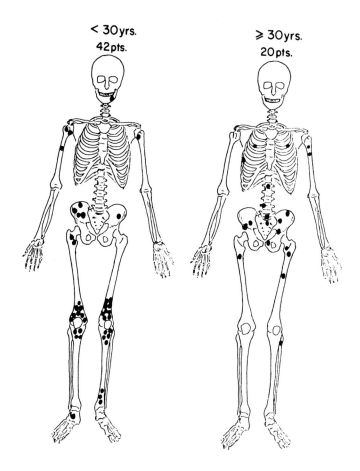

Fig. 2. Osteosarcoma. Primary site of involvement.

Thus, in our experience, radical irradiation offered only temporary growth restraint to these patients, since in all patients there was either failure of control of recurrence at the primary site.

TABLE 1. Osteosarcoma. Duration and Degree of Response to Irradiation

Response	No. of Patients	Duration (Mths)		
		Range	Mean	Median
CR	3	3-6	4	4
PR	17	1-9	5.5	5.5
NR	7	0	0	0

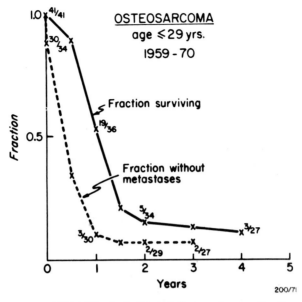

Fig. 3. Osteosarcoma. 1959-1970. Crude Survival Curve and proportion free of metastatic disease.

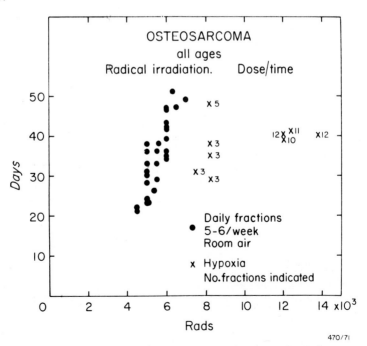

Fig. 4. Osteosarcoma. Dose/time relationships for primary irradiation.

The morbidity associated with a reactive primary was severe. Pain, limitation of joint movement, and the danger of fracture in a weight-bearing bone, were the factors that markedly limited the activity of these patients. Only three of 17 patients with a lower limb tumour had an initially good functional result, and these had recurred within three months.

For the radically irradiated patient, the mean time to recurrence was 3.6 months, to the development of secondaries 4.5 months, and to death 13 months. Pulmonary metastases did not usually produce major functional impairment until the last few weeks of life, so that symptoms associated with the primary site were dominant for most patients.

What then were the indications for ablation of a limb? Twenty-two patients with the primary site in the arm or leg were radically irradiated and followed for at least six months. Each developed either primary recurrence or metastases or both, during the six-month follow-up period. Elective surgical ablation at six months was therefore appropriate for none. Ablative surgery was carried out in 12 of the 22 patients. In eight, the indication was recurrence at the primary tumour and in the absence of metastatic disease. Three other patients required palliative amputation after the development of pulmonary metastases, and in one patient an elective amputation was performed at two months, whilst the patient was asymptomatic and the tumour clinically under control, but pathological examination demonstrated gross tumour.

The retention of a painful limb of limited use was associated with the early onset of systemic symptoms, particularly loss of appetite and well-being. There was increased use of analgesics, and frequently depression, for the failure of tumour control in a peripheral bone tumour is as evident to the patient as to the physician. In this situation palliative amputation is better undertaken early than late.

In summary, I emphasize that our original premise was that radical irradiation is indicated in the management of peripheral osteosarcoma only if good local palliation is achieved, so that amputation may be avoided in those patients metastasizing early. It is clear that in our experience these conditions were not met. We have therefore come to believe that immediate surgical ablation is indicated in osteosarcoma, and that radical irradiation should be reserved for the minority of patients where the site of the tumour makes resection impractical.

Ewing's Sarcoma

In sharp contrast to osteosarcoma, Ewing's sarcoma as a rule responds rapidly and completely to local irradiation and there is prompt recovery of any functional disturbance.

It is important that the tissue volume irradiated be adequately large. For limb tumours the whole of the involved bone, together with all its associated soft tissues, is included in the irradiated volume. For tumours involving trunk bones, particularly the pelvic bones, a full radiological investigation, which will often include angiography, is obligatory, for these tumours are often much larger than indicated by palpation alone. We irradiate the chosen volume to a minimum tumour dose of 5,000 rads in five weeks. By the completion of such a course, the response is usually complete.

The cure rate in this tumour remains modest because metastases, chiefly to lung and bone, occur early and frequently. The cure rate is the same whether the primary treatment is by irradiation or surgery. Since response to irradiation is rapid and complete, this is the preferred treatment in that unnecessary amputations are avoided.

In recent years, the attention in this tumour has been focused on systemic management of the metastatic component of the disease, for it has long been recognized that good objective remissions can be obtained with chemotherapy, particularly with Cyclophosphamide and Vincristine.

The results obtained at The Princess Margaret Hospital and the Hospital for Sick Children in Toronto are shown (Fig.5). For 31 patients treated from 1929 to 1959, the primary was most often irradiated but with no uniformity of dose or volume. Amputation was occasionally performed. Little active treatment was given in the metastatic phase of the disease. These patients serve as a base-line for our subsequent experience. Sixty-eight percent of these patients died in the

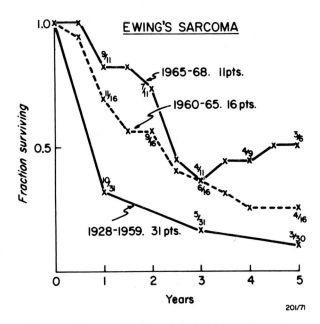

Fig. 5. Ewing's Sarcoma. Crude survival related to year of diagnosis.

first year after diagnosis. Three of the 30, 10% were cured. From 1960-1965, 16 patients without demonstrable secondaries at diagnosis were treated by irradiation. The volume irradiated was relatively standardized and a dose in the range 4,500-6,000 rads in three to six weeks were employed. Metastatic disease was managed by local irradiation, 2,000 rads in four to six days combined with chemotherapy, most often using Cyclophosphamide 2.5 mgm per kilogram per day, P.O. An improvement in the five-year survival rate was seen in that four of 16 survived. There was also marked improvement in the control of the early metastatic phase of the disease with approximately 2/3 of the patients being alive at one year.

In 1965 we commenced a trial of adjuvant total body irradiation in Ewing's sarcoma. This was given electively, with a single dose of 300 rads following radical irradiation of the primary tumour. This was combined with more aggressive irradiation and chemotherapy in the later overt metastatic phase of the disease. There may well have been further improvement in our results, but the numbers are too small to be sure.

It is particularly encouraging that two of our three five-year survivors from this period had single sites of metastatic disease apparent at the time of initial diagnosis. This is the first time in our experience that such patients have obtained prolonged survival.

Of the 27 patients treated since 1960, only one has required amputation for recurrence of the primary tumour, whilst still free of metastatic disease. Recurrence at the primary tumour site during the metastatic phase of the disease can usually be satisfactorily managed by palliative irradiation and chemotherapy. Palliative amputation has not been necessary.

Since 1970, we have increased our elective systemic therapy to include a 12-month course of alternating Cyclophosphamide and Vincristine for it has become evident that in this disease the onset of the overt metastatic phase may be at least suppressed by such therapy for prolonged periods, though we must wait longer to know whether the cure rate will be improved.

In summary and in contrast to osteosarcoma, Ewing's sarcoma responds well to both irradiation and chemotherapy appropriately applied, and there is some promise that energetic systemic therapy of occult metastatic disease may improve the modest cure rate.

References

1. Jenkin, R. D. T.: Ewing's Sarcoma. A Study of Treatment Methods. *Clin. Radio.* 17:97-106, April, 1966.
2. Jenkin, R. D. T., Rider, W. D., and Sonley, M. J.: Ewing's Sarcoma. A Trial of Adjuvant Total-Body Irradiation. *Radiology,* 96. 1:151-155, July, 1970.
3. Jenkin, R. D. T., Allt, W. E. C., Fitzpatrick, P. J.: Osteosarcoma. An Assessment of Management with Particular Reference to Primary Irradiation and Selective Delayed Amputation. *Cancer* (In Press).

Management of Ewing's Tumor in Children

Lucius F. Sinks, M.D. and Arnold I. Freeman, M.D.

Introduction

In 1921, Ewing described a bone tumor comprised of small round cells which he termed a "diffuse endothelioma of bone" because he believed that the tumor was of endothelial origin.[3] To this date controversy has raged over the origin of this tumor. In particular, differentiation between Ewing's tumor and primary reticulum cell sarcoma of bone has been difficult.

The primary treatment for Ewing's sarcoma has been either radiotherapy to the involved area, or surgery. The results in either case have been poor. Falk's review of the literature on 987 cases yielded only an 8%, five year cure rate.[4] Recently, adjuvant chemotherapy, along with primary treatment of the involved bone, has suggested a considerable improvement in the cure rate.[6,8,9]

The present report reviews the treatment and results to date of 20 cases of Ewing's tumor in children treated at Roswell Park Memorial Institute between 1954 and 1970.

Clinical Material

We reviewed the charts of 20 pediatric patients who were treated from 1954 to 1970.

Age and Sex

Patients, at presentation, varied in age from 18 months to 17 years. Seven of the patients were under ten years of age. There was a slight male preponderance with 11 males to 9 females.

Presentation

All 20 patients presented with some discomfort related to the involved bone. In addition, there was swelling related to this area in the majority of patients. The breakdown of the site of initial involvement is as follows: femor 6, fibula 3,

Lucius F. Sinks, M.D. *and* Arnold I. Freeman, M.D., *Department of Pediatrics, Roswell Park Memorial Institute, Buffalo, New York.*

This work was supported in part by CA-07918.

radius 3, ileum 3, scapula 2, humerus 2, and vertebra 1. Fourteen patients presented with involvement of the long bones, and the remainder presented with tumor in the bones of the trunk. Three patients had metastatic disease in the lungs at presentation.

Primary Treatment

No Treatment

In Cases 1 and 2, the family refused treatment. Note, in Case 1 the patient received only a half dose of nitrogen mustard, then further treatment was refused. Both cases died from their disease.

Surgery

Amputation was performed in Cases 3 to 5. The three cases all died from their tumor.

Radiotherapy

Out of 20 patients, six patients received radiation therapy only as primary treatment (Cases 6 to 11). There is no information available in one patient, Case 6. In the patients treated at Roswell Park Memorial Institute, the entire bone was included in the irradiated fields. The megavoltage equipment used in patients was CO^{60} with source skin distance of 80 cms and half value layer of 10.4 mm Pb. All patients were treated with anterior and posterior fields and the tumor dose was calculated at the midline. In patients initially treated elsewhere, 250 KVP as well as CO^{60} was employed.

Radiotherapy and Chemotherapy

Radiotherapy plus chemotherapy were employed as the initial treatment in nine cases (Cases 12 to 20). The radiotherapy in these cases was essentially the same as that which was used above, when it was used alone. In recent years, adjuvant chemotherapy has generally consisted of cyclophosphamide (Cytoxan) 300 mgm/m² i.v. weekly for 6 weeks, followed by a six week rest. The cycle is repeated for approximately one year. Among these nine cases, three are potential cures (Cases 13, 16, and 17) with disease-free intervals of 11 years, 38 months, and 36 months, respectively. Case 13 is of particular interest since she presented with metastatic disease in her lungs. The disease responded to radiotherapy and Cytoxan without recurrence for over 12 years. Case 15 is also noteworthy. At initial presentation he had metastatic disease in his lungs and was treated with radiotherapy to his primary lung lesion, and BCNU (3-bis-(2 Chlorethyl)-1-Nitrosourea). The lung lesion shrank by approximately 75%, but did not disappear, remaining static for approximately three years. Surgical intervention was avoided during this period because x-ray suggested the presence of a fluid-filled cyst. However, when this lesion began to expand after three years, thoracotomy was performed which revealed Ewing's tumor. The patient was retreated with BCNU at intervals for 12 months and shows no evidence of disease two years later. It is felt that he may be another potential cure, although on the other hand, the chemotherapy may be just delaying the Ewing's sarcoma from reappearing.

Recurrent Disease

Reactivation

Reactivation of the Ewing's tumor at the primary site occurred in three instances prior to metastasis (Cases 10, 12, and 14), and in two instances simultaneous with metastasis (Cases 8 and 19) (see Table 1). The radiation dosage varied from 3900 to 5000 rads in these cases. It occurred in two patients receiving radiotherapy and chemotherapy.

TABLE 1. Reactivation of the Primary Site

Case Number	8	10	12	14	19
Radiation dose (primary) (rads)	3900	4000	3000	4000	5000
Site of Primary	femur	ileum	scapula	fibula	vertebra
Time to Reactivation	3 mon.	8	6 mon.	16	6
Reactivation simultaneous with metastasis	+				+
Reactivation prior to metastasis		+	+	+	
Site of first metastasis	lungs	lungs		lungs	lungs
Time to metastasis after reactivation		5 mon.	?	3 mon.	

Distant Metastasis

Distant metastasis was the first evidence of recurrent disease in nine patients. The time to metastasis varied from one month to 16 months, with a median of three months, and an average of 7.1 months. Metastases were first noted in the lungs in six cases, and in the bone in one case, the lung and bone simultaneously in one case, and in the soft tissue of the orbit in one case.

Discussion

Classical treatment with either surgery or radiotherapy, aimed at ablation of primary Ewing's tumor, has proved disappointing. Either method has yielded a similarly low cure rate (see Table 3).

Classical treatment may fail because subclinical micrometastasis are likely present at the time of initial diagnosis and treatment. To effect a cure, these micrometastases must be irradicated. Total body irradiation, along with the treatment of the primary site, has been attempted as one approach to cure.[7,11] Of 11 patients treated in this fashion, six were apparently free of disease at a

TABLE 2. Historical Comparison of the Different
Treatments of Ewing's Sarcoma

Treatment	Investigator	No. of Patients	Results
Radiotherapy	Wang and Schultz (15)	22	4 5-year survivors
Radiotherapy	Suit (14)	23	1 5-year survivor
Surgery	Geschickter and Copeland (5)	37	7 5-year survivors
Surgery	Dahlin (2)	19	5 5-year survivors
Radiotherapy and Surgery	Geschickter and Copeland (5)	22	3 5-year survivors
Radiotherapy and Surgery	Dahlin (2)	21	4 5-year survivors
Radiotherapy and Chemotherapy	Phillips and Higinbotham (13)	54*	13 5-year survivors
Radiotherapy and Chemotherapy	Hustu et al (6)	5	5 disease free at 1+ years
Radiotherapy and Chemotherapy	Johnson et al (8)	24**	7 disease free from 6+ to 63+ months
Radiotherapy to primary + total body irradiation	Jenkins and Melburn (11)	11	6 disease free at 2 years

*Of these, 39 patients had localized disease at presentation and were treated with intent to cure.

**Of these, 24 patients, 7 presented with metastatic disease and 3 have been followed less than 6 months and are not evaluated in the disease-free status.

two year follow-up. A second approach consists of the primary treatment and adjuvant chemotherapy.[6,8,9,13] We favor the second approach because toxicity can be more easily monitored by alteration of drug dosage, and repeated chemotherapy courses can be readily given. In the treatment of a primary localized Ewings, Hustu used localized irradiation and adjuvant chemotherapy in five patients. None showed recurrent or metastatic disease in a follow-up of one year later or longer.[6] Johnson used a similar program in 14 patients with primary localized Ewings. Seven patients have been disease-free from 6 plus to 63 plus months.[8] Phillips used radiotherapy plus various chemotherapeutic adjuvants. Thirteen of his 39 patients with localized Ewings survived for five years.[13]

In our own series, nine patients received primary adjuvant chemotherapy along with radiotherapy. At present, the chemotherapy regimen at Roswell Park, in cases seen early in their disease, consists of Cytoxan 300 mgm/m^2 i.v./wk. for six weeks followed by a six week rest. The entire cycle is then repeated for a total period of one year and then chemotherapy is stopped. The patient continues to be observed closely with chest x-rays monthly, and x-rays of the primary site approximately every two to three months. Three are disease-free, and one additional case may be a potential cure, although it is too early to be certain. None of the twenty cases was cured without chemotherapy during the initial treatment. It should be noted that metastatic disease or reactivation of the primary site manifested themselves early in the course of disease. The longest time from initial therapy to metastasis was 16 months. It is recognized that metastasis in Ewings may be detected late in the course of the disease; however, this appears to be uncommon, and a disease-free state of two years appears to indicate an excellent chance of cure. Since metastases usually manifest themselves during the first 12 to 18 months, it is speculated that the chemotherapy should be given for approximately the same period of time.

Unlike the recent report of Marsa and Johnson,[10] brain metastasis were not the site of primary metastatic disease, but did occur on occasion in terminal disease. This finding was consistent even when the patients received adjuvant chemotherapy.

Particularly distressing in the present report are five cases in whom the primary site of the disease was reactivated: three cases prior to distant metastasis and two cases simultaneous with metastasis. Suit[14] and Jenkins[17] have noted similar cases in their reports. These findings imply that tumor cells were not completely irradicated from the primary site, and that they acted as a nidus to spread tumor throughout the body. In our patients, from 3900 to 5000 rads tumor dose has been used. To combat reactivation, two approaches are feasible: amputation, when feasible, or an increase in the midline dosage of radiotherapy to approximately 6000 rads in 30 fractions over six weeks. The latter approach appears to be more attractive, at present, since it saves a limb, and since historically, surgery offers no clear-cut advantage over radiotherapy (see Table 2)[14]; in fact, this latter approach is now being used at Roswell Park. However, should reactivation of the primary site occur after radiotherapy, and without distant metastasis, prompt amputation of the primary lesion, if feasible, and a change in the chemotherapeutic agents should be instituted. These measures appear to be indicated on the basis that the tumor is still localized and thus curable.

Since Ewings is a rare tumor, however, with an estimated 150 new cases seen in the United States annually,[12] a national study with randomized allocation is necessary, if we are to answer definitely which primary treatment is best.

Summary

Twenty pediatric patients with Ewing's tumor seen at Roswell Park Memorial Institute from 1954 to 1970 have been analyzed. Four patients are free of disease for over three years.

At the initial treatment, these four patients were all treated with radiotherapy to the primary tumor and adjuvant chemotherapy. Nine of the 20 patients were treated in this fashion. It is felt that the chemotherapy is irradicating the subclinical micrometastasis and thus effecting a cure.

Five cases with reactivation of their primary sites prior to or simultaneous with metastasis were noted, indicating incomplete sterilization of tumor by present radiotherapeutic techniques and suggesting that more aggressive therapy be directed to the primary site along with the systemic chemotherapy.

References

1. Boyer, C. W., Jr., Brickner, T. J., Jr., Perry, R. H.: Ewing's sarcoma: Case against surgery. *Cancer* 20:1602-1606, Oct. 1967.
2. Dahlin, D., Coventry, M. and Scanlon, P.: Ewing's sarcoma. *J. Bone Surg.* 43-A (2):185-192, 1961.
3. Ewing, J.: Diffuse endothelioma of bone. *Proc. N. Y. Path. Soc.* 21:17-24, 1921.
4. Falk, S., Alpert, M.: Five-year survival of patients with Ewing's sarcoma. *Surg. Gynec. Obstet.* 124:319-324, Feb. 1967.
5. Geschickter, C. and Copeland, M.: *Tumors of Bone* 3rd Edition. Philadelphia: J. B. Lippincott, 1949, pp. 287-434.
6. Hustu, H. O., Holton, C., James, D., Jr., et al: Treatment of Ewing's sarcoma with concurrent radiotherapy and chemotherapy. *J. Pediat.* 73:249-251, August 1968.
7. Jenkin, R. D. T.: Ewing's sarcoma: Study of treatment methods. *Clin. Radiol.* 17:97-106, April 1966.
8. Johnson, R. and Humphreys, S. R.: Past failures and future possibilities in Ewing's sarcoma: Experimental and preliminary clinical results. *Cancer* 23:161-166, Jan., 1969.
9. Johnson, R. E., Senyszyn, J. J., Rabson, A. S. and Peterson, K. A.: Treatment of Ewing's sarcoma with local irradiation and systemic chemotherapy. A progress report. *Radiology* 95:195-197, April, 1970.
10. Marsa, G. W. and Johnson, R. E.: Altered pattern of metastasis following treatment of Ewing's sarcoma with radiotherapy and adjuvant chemotherapy. *Cancer* 27:1051, 1971.
11. Milburn, L. F., O'Grady, L., Hendrickson, F. R.: Radical radiation therapy and total body irradiation in the treatment of Ewing's sarcoma. *Cancer* 22:919-925, Nov. 1968.
12. Miller, R. W.: Fifty-two forms of childhood cancer: United States mortality experience, 1960-1966. *J. Pediat.* 75:685-689, 1969.
13. Phillips, R. F. and Higinbotham, N. L.: The curability of Ewing's endothelioma of bone in children. *J. Pediat.* 70:391-397, 1967.
14. Suit, H.: Ewing's sarcoma: Treatment by radiation therapy. In: *Tumor of bone and soft tissue* Chicago: Yearbook, Medical Publishers, Inc., 1965, pp. 191-200.
15. Wang, C. and Schultz, M.: Ewing's sarcoma, *N.E.J.M.* 288:571-576, 1953.

Retinoblastoma

Carmine Bedotto, M.D.

Introduction

Retinoblastoma is the most common ocular tumor of childhood.[1] It is a highly malignant tumor which usually manifests itself within the first two years of life, and is transmittable by an autosomal dominant gene with 80-95% penetrance.[1,2] It thus can occur in a familial pattern or appear sporadically. Sporadic cases are felt to arise from phenocopies and somatic mutations which are unilateral and not transmittable or germ cell mutations which can be unilateral or bilateral and will be transmittable.[2] Apparent sporadic cases can also result from parents who possess the gene but are phenotypically normal due to non-penetrance. These cases are usually bilateral but rarely can affect only one eye.

The tumor arises in the nuclear layers of the retina[1] in one or more independent foci which expand within the retina and later can fill the vitreous cavity (Fig. 1, 2). It can also invade the choroid, but the retinal pigment epithelium and Bruch's Membrane act as relative barriers. Eventually, the tumor can perforate the eye, but the most common route of extraocular spread is through the optic nerve into the subarachnoid space (Fig. 3). The prognosis is significantly lessened if the tumor has invaded the nerve beyond the lamina cribrosa.[1]

Evaluation

The proper evaluation of these children is extremely important. General anesthesia is necessary so that one can use the binocular indirect ophthalmoscope with scleral depression to visualize the entire retina. Only in this way can one detect tiny tumors especially when they lie anterior to the equator.

The presenting symptoms in a series of cases from London are shown in Table 1.[3] Leucokoria and squint are the most common symptoms while a painful, glaucomatous eye possibly with a hyphema occurs when the tumor fills the globe. The children seen without symptoms had a positive family history and

Carmine Bedotto, M.D., *Bascom Palmer Eye Institute, University of Miami School of Medicine, Department of Ophthalmology, Miami, Florida.*

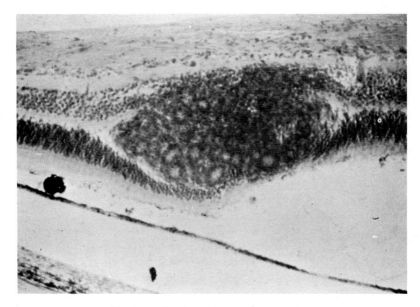

Fig. 1. Small retinoblastoma arising in retina.

were routinely examined within the first three to four weeks after birth. The typical appearance of retinoblastoma is a slightly pink, solid mass which may show flecks of calcium as it enlarged. The retinal vessels which serve the tumor may be dilated (Fig. 4, 6).

Treatment

The modalities of therapy which are utilized today are listed in Table 2. The treatment of retinoblastoma has changed considerably since enucleation offered the only hope. Foster-Moore and Stallard[4,5] utilized radon seeds and Martin and Reese[6] administered external kilovoltage radiation in early attempts to eradicate retinoblastomas while saving some vision. Stallard[7] used pathological evidence

TABLE 1. Presenting Symptoms of Retinoblastoma

Symptoms	Cases
White pupil reflex	44
Squint	28
Painful red eye	6
Hyphema	2
Combination of several	10
None	13
Not recorded	36

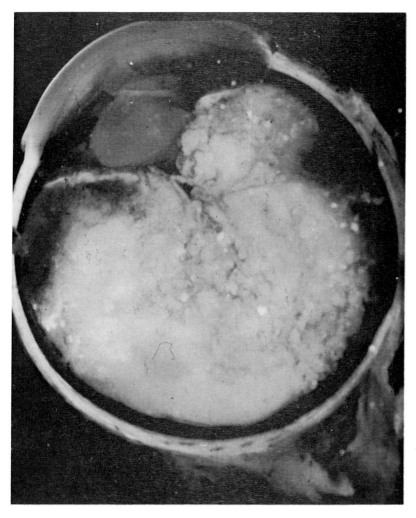

Fig. 2. Massive retinoblastoma filling vitreous cavity.

TABLE 2. Treatment of Retinoblastoma

Radiation
  a. External Radiation Therapy
  b. Focal Radiation with Cobalt 60 Applicators
Photocoagulation
Cryotherapy
Chemotherapy-TEM
Enucleation

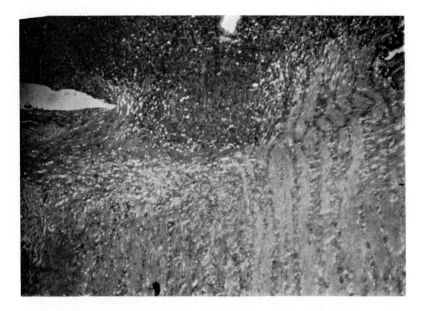

Fig. 3. Retinoblastoma invading optic nerve to level of lamina cribrosa.

and Reese et.al.[8] developed clinical data to independently arrive at 3,500 R as the therapeutic dose of radiation. The older methods of external irradiation have now been replaced with external supervoltage therapy which allows us to treat the tumor with a minimum of radiation damage to normal structures.[3,9,10]

External supervoltage therapy in London where I studied was devised by I. G. Williams[11] whose paper follows so I will limit this discussion to the indications for this type of therapy.

Large tumors over 10 to 13 mm in diameter, tumors of any size near the disc or macula, or tumors with vitreous seeding are treated with cobalt beam through an anterior field. The temporal approach with the linear accelerator or betatron in an only eye with a posterior pole tumor can also be used to spare the lens from radiation. The external therapy does not appear to damage the normal retina or optic nerve, but electrical retinal function studies must be performed as large numbers of these children become older. At present we know that many retain normal vision if the tumor did not damage the macula (Fig. 4 to 7). A cataract of varying degree always develops when the anterior field is used for the therapy: when they are severe enough to reduce vision or prevent examination of the fundus, they can be removed by conventional aspiration methods (Fig. 8).

One solitary tumor or groups of tumors less than 10 mm diameter can be treated by suturing a cobalt 60 applicator to the sclera under the tumor. They were designed by Innes and Stallard[12,13] to deliver a continuous dose of therapeutic irradiation over six to seven days without radiating the entire eye.

These applicators destroy a rim of normal tissue around the tumor so they cannot be used near the nerve or macula without jeopardizing vision. They are also useful for treating recurrent tumor after external therapy when a second dose of radiation to the entire eye may produce severe complications. Because of the multifocal nature of retinoblastoma, new primary tumors occur after focal methods of treatment in 20% of the cases so this must be considered in the follow-up.[3]

Photocoagulation[14] and cryotherapy[15,16] are useful for treating small tumors under 4 mm in diameter again away from the optic disc and macula as surrounding normal tissue is destroyed. These methods are especially useful in treating recurrences post irradiation.

Triethylene melamine (TEM) is a chemotherapeutic drug used at Columbia Presbyterian Hospital[17,18] for tumors over 15 mm in diameter always in

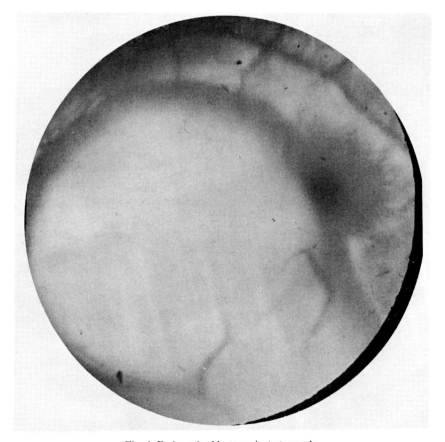

Fig. 4. Early retinoblastoma just at macula.

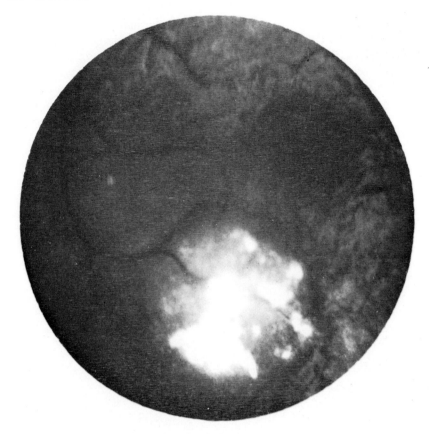

Fig. 5. Same as Figure 4 post cobalt beam therapy. Note normal macula appearance and inactive calcified tumor debris.

conjunction with external radiation therapy. The intracarotid administration has proven very helpful in controlling these large tumors.

Table 3 shows the results obtained in London in all cases treated between 1960 and 1970. 132 eyes were treated by all methods, 108 eyes have been saved at the time the paper was written.[3] Of the 24 eyes lost, 22 were enucleated post treatment while 2 eyes contained active recurrences but were not removed as the children had orbital recurrences from the initially enucleated fellow eye and were near death. Analysis of the 24 eyes removed post treatment reveals that 13 had active recurrences which could not be controlled and 9 had blind, painful eyes from radiation complications. Better understanding of the eyes' tolerance for radiation in recent years has reduced this problem somewhat during the later period of the study.[3]

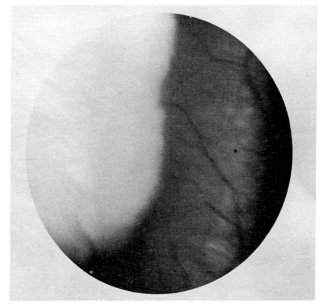

Fig. 6. Larger retinoblastoma.

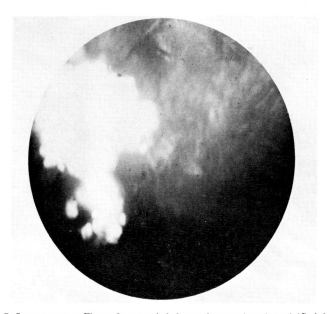

Fig. 7. Same tumor as Figure 6 post cobalt beam therapy, inactive calcified debris.

TABLE 3. Results of Eyes Treated

Total eyes treated	132
Eyes active but not enucleated	2
Eyes enucleated post treatment	22
For active tumor	13
For radiation complications	9

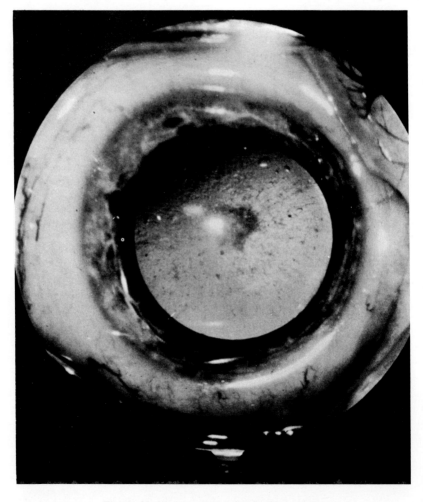

Fig. 8. Moderately advanced radiation cataract.

Retinoblastoma has been classified Class 1 to V[1] and recent evidence shows that successful control of small tumors is about 90% while even extensive ones can often be arrested.[3,9,10,17] When the visual function of an eye is lost due to tumor or radiation the eye should be enucleated. Death usually occurs by central nervous system spread via the optic nerve or less frequently through blood born metastases which significantly rise once the choroid has been invaded.[1]

Genetic Counselling

Genetic counselling of the parents and cured patients is important and is summarized in Table 4.[2,19] The important aspect is to advise the people that all newborn children should be examined within the first month of life.

TABLE 4. Genetic Counselling in Retinoblastoma

1. To Parents
   a. Sporadic case with no FH – 6% chance another child will get a retinoblastoma
   b. FH (+) – 40% + chance another child will get a retinoblastoma

2. To Patient
   a. Sporadic case with no FH – 25% chance it will be the transmittable type
   b. FH + – 40% + chance each child can get a retinoblastoma

References

1. Reese, A. B.: *Tumors of the Eye* 2nd ed. New York:Hoeber.
2. Francois, J. and VanLeuven, M. T. M.: in *Ocular and Adnexal Tumors,* (ed.) M. Boniuk. St. Louis:Mosby, p. 123, 1964.
3. Bedford, M. A., Bedotto, C., and MacFaul, P. A.: Retinoblastoma, *British Journ. Ophthal.* 55:19, 1971.
4. Moore, R. Foster: *Proc. Roy. Sec. Med.* 22:951, 1929.
5. Moore, R. Foster, Stallard, H. B. and Milner, J. G.: *Brit. Journ. Ophthal.* 15:673, 1931.
6. Martin, H. E., and Reese, A. B.: *Arch. Ophth* 16:733, 1936.
7. Stallard, H. B.: *Brit. Med. Journ.* 2:962, 1936.
8. Reese, A. B., Hyman, G. A., Tapley, N. DeV., and Forrest, A. W.: *A.M.A. Arch. Ophth.* 60:897, 1958.
9. Ellsworth, R. M.: *Am. J. Ophthal.* 66:49, 1968.
10. Cassady, J. P., Sagerman, R. H., Tretter, P., and Ellsworth, R. M.: *Radiology* 93:405, 1969.
11. Skaggs, D. B. L., and Williams, I. G.: *Clin Radiol.* 17:169, 1966.
12. Innes, G. S.: in *Ocular and Adnexal Tumors* (ed.) M. Boniuk, St. Louis:Mosby, p. 142.
13. Stallard, H. B.: *Trans. Ophthal. Soc. U. K.* 82:473, 1962.
14. Hopping, W., and Meyer-Schwicketath, G.: in *Ocular and Adnexal Tumors* (ed.) M. Boniuk, St. Louis:Mosby, p. 192.
15. Lincoff, H., McLean, J., and Long, R.: *Am. J. Ophthal.* 63:389, 1967.
16. Rubin, M. L., *Am. J. Ophthal.* 66:870, 1968.
17. Hyman, J. A., Ellsworth, R. M., Feind, D. R. and Tretter, P.: *Arch. Ophth.* 80:744, 1968.
18. Gillette, R., and Bodenstein, D.: *J. Exp. Zool.* 103:1, 1946.
19. Banks, L. N.: *Brit. Journ. Ophth.* 53:212, 1969.

Bilateral Retinoblastoma

I. G. Williams, M.B., F.R.C.S., F.F.R.

This discussion concerns us with the treatment of children affected with bilateral retinoblastoma, i.e. a highly malignant cancer affecting both eyes of a very young child. The problems are perplexing, fascinating medically, and tragic emotionally. We are discussing the child where in 99% one eye has been removed, and the tumour in the remaining eye is so extensive as to make it unsuitable for treatment by very localized therapy. The aim is twofold:

1. To save life, for it is a malignant cancer.

2. To preserve some degree of vision without prejudice to life.

The alternative to radiotherapy compatible with survival is removal of both eyes and with this total blindness. Retinoblastoma is a congenital tumour commoner in the white than the coloured races. The eyes may be full of neoplasm at birth. Most are diagnosed in the first 12 months of life, 70% in the first three years, diminishing to 6% after the age of six years. It is often noted by the mother, the cat's eye reflex − a greyish white reflex to light behind the pupil. When this is evident the growth involves more than half the retina, the remainder being either partially or totally detached. The tumour occurs sporadically, or with a familial incidence, and it can affect one or both eyes.

Bilateral disease is due to two distinct primary tumours, and the growth is more advanced and larger in one eye than the other. The incidence is about one-third of all cases. Bilateral disease is commoner in (1) those detected in the first year of life, and (2) those with a family history. The children of parents with one eye affected, if they develop the tumour do so most often in both eyes. Although they may coincide, there may be a time interval between the appearance of the tumour in the first and then the second eye. Whilst this is oftenest within 12 months, there is a patient on record where this interval was 11 years. Indeed in my own experience I had one of 12 years.

The tendency for tumours to be bilateral increases with each generation, and this emphasizes the importance of frequent periodic examinations. For accurate examination, the pupil must be fully dilated, the tumour or tumours are then seen as granular cheesy flocculent masses with associated fine blood vessels. Single or multiple islands may be present.

I. G. Williams, M.B., F.R.C.S., F.F.R., *Consultant Radiotherapist, St. Bartholomew's Hospital And The Hospital For Sick Children, Great Ormond Street, London, England.*

The classical treatment of unilateral disease is enucleation of the eye, the result here depending entirely upon whether there is extension along the optic nerve of the excised eye. A long part of the nerve must be obtained in order to place the section behind the point of nerve invasion. If this is not so 95% will develop orbital recurrences within 18 months. If the nerve is not invaded, prognosis will depend upon whether a tumour develops in the other eye.

Whilst there may be agreement, between surgeon and parents, as to the indications for enucleation in unilateral disease, when the tumours are bilateral, considerations are much more difficult. In these, the disease is more advanced in one eye than the other. There is no purpose in keeping an eye which is blind, or where the effects of treatment results in blindness, but it is justifiable to attempt to conserve vision in the less affected eye if this can be done without jeopardising the life of the patient.

Radiotherapy

Large or multiple tumours are unsuitable for treatment by radioactive discs, light coagulation, or other local therapy. In these the heavy local irradiation in 9-12 months results in vitreous haemorrhage or uveitis, and this will spoil the visual results. Tumours at the edge of the optic disc or at the ora serrata are difficult to cover, and inadequate coverage will result in failure. The conditions prone to result in failure of localised treatment depend upon the site, size, and local spread of the neoplasm, and on dissemination by seeding into the vitreous, and forwards into the gutters between the ciliary processes.

Very small tumours can, of course, be dealt with by light coagulation or radioactive discs. If these are contraindicated we use external irradiation with megavoltage Cobalt 60 beam. The whole vitreous and whole retina are irradiated through an anterior field 2 X 3 cms or 3 X 4 cms. We believe that the whole vitreous and the entire retina must be irradiated, and this implies that the whole eye must be included. Through an anterior field the whole eye can be included in the 80% isodose. Note also the 30% dose on the surface of the cornea. The simplest is a direct anterior field.

Lateral fields, in trying to spare the lens, may also spare some retina and some vitreous. Cataract is the main complication and we feel it is a small penalty to pay and indeed can be dealt with. Blindness is due much more to scarring of tumours, at or near the macula after treatment; this is outside our control. Operations for cataract in these children are no more difficult than in other causes of cataract, and the method of aspiration evolved and developed in the U.S.A. is atraumatic and they are only an in-patient for two days.

Technique

The technique we employ is as follows:

In small babies, and most are under the age of one year, an anaesthetic is essential. We use Ketalar and because of this we fractionate three times a week

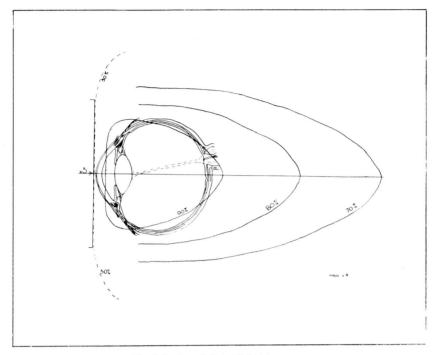

Fig. 1. Isodose Cobalt 60 3 × 4 cms.

giving 300-350 rads applied per treatment to a total dose of 3500-4000 rads in 3-4 weeks. At 80% isodose the whole eye gets 3200 rads — a dose we know to be curative in other embryonic tumours such as neuroblastoma and seminoma.

Reactions and Complications

Local reactions are slight, there is minimal reddening of the eyelids and conjunctiva, and the eyebrows may depilate. The various anatomical components of the eye exhibit a wide range of radiosensitivity well within the margin of tolerance of this dose. I cannot discuss these now apart from the lens. Keeping the eye open does *not* seem to affect local reactions and we do not deliberately keep the lids apart.

Radiation Cataract

This is the most important complication which develops to some extent and of some degree in all our patients. The lens receives a dose of between 1500-3500 rads.

The children are admitted every four to six weeks in the first year after treatment and every six to eight weeks in the second year. We have been doing this for over ten years, but in the last five years have been able to document the changes photographically with the KOWA fundus camera. An inactive tumour looks hard and solid, white in colour and with speckled or gross calcification. An

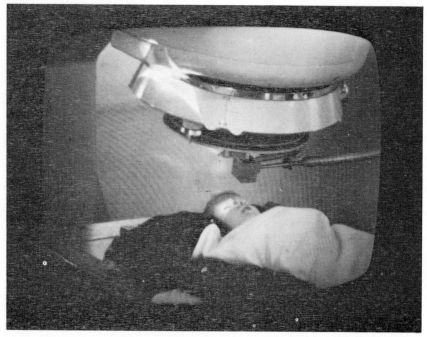

Fig. 2. Television view of child under treatment with Ketalar anaesthesia. Note lead block on medial side to protect nasal bone and pituitary.

active tumour stimulates the proliferation of fine blood vessels. If the surface of a nodule is coagulated with a light beam in an active tumour, vessels appear.

We have not found V.M.A. estimations of any value as an indication or index of activity.

The dose which produces a cataract is very variable. Some of the Hiroshima victims developed a cataract without any other sign of radiation injury. Doses as low as 200 rads have been cataractogenic and the range is said to be between 800-1200 rads. This will produce a cataract after a latent period of 1-12 years. Merrian and Focht (1957) in their now classical report based on animal work, state that young lenses are more sensitive than the adult. In their analysis lenses of children below the age of one year showed a higher incidence and more rapid development. Over the age of one year, the lenses of children appear to have the same sensitivity as the adult. Lens fibres are produced by division of cells lying at the lens equator. Behind this line the cells are non-nucleated. The young growing equatorial cells are very sensitive and damage to these results in abnormal lens fibres, some nucleated migrating towards the posterior pole where they remain throughout life. The sum of the damage produces characteristic lens opacities. They can be progressive until complete, or small and multiple giving a stippled lens. They may progress to a certain size and then remain stationary or advance very, very slowly.

We (Bedford and MacFaul) classify cataract into four main types:

1. *Doughnut type:* Develops about two years after irradiation. This is the classical large type following direct irradiation of the eye as described. Surgical treatment is possible and gives good results.

2. *Posterior subcapsular:* The posterior part of the lens becomes entirely opacified, and this also occurs after direct irradiation.

3. *Sectoral opacities:* Localised non-progressive opacities which follow the application of radioactive plaques.

4. *Complete and total cataract:* Appears two to three years after exposure of the whole eye to large doses, i.e. as a consequence of the treatment of tumours of the nasal sinuses.

Results

1962-1969

Total reviewed	$-$ 65
Bilateral	$-$ 57 (2nd eye $-$ 1st having been removed)
Died from disease	$-$ 4 (Extension back 3, generalised mets. 1)
Alive with some useful vision and no active tumour	$-$ 37 (65%)
(Minimal follow-up is two years)	
Alive eye retained, disease static. Blind.	
(Very slight perception of light)	$-$ 2
Eye subsequently excised	$-$ 14
Complete retinal detachment	$-$ 2
Failure to eradicate tumour	$-$ 12

Cataract

Occurred in all cases	$-$ 100%
Doughnut type in 13	$-$ 20%

(Treated by aspiration and most have 20/20 vision.)

Remainder nonprogressive. Stippled. Varying extent

$$5/20 - 20/20$$

Although the radiotherapy technique of a single applied field to the eye is simple and easy, the assessment of the suitability for this treatment, the interpretation of the effects and response requires long experience and guidance. I would urge any radiotherapist who undertakes this to do it hand in hand with an experienced specialist in eye diseases, but I can assure you that a successful result is one of the most gratifying experiences in radiotherapy.

References

1. MacFaul, P. A. and Bedford, M. A.: Ocular complications after Therapeutic Irradiation. *Brit. J. Ophthalmol.* 54, 4:237-247, 1970.
2. Skeggs, D. B. L. and Williams, I. G.: The treatment of advanced retinoblastoma by means of external irradiation combined with chemotherapy. *Clinical Radiology,* XVII 2:169-172, 1966.
3. Williams, I. G.: *Let there be Light.* Proceedings of the Royal Society of Medicine 60, 2:189-196, 1967.

Radiotherapy of Chiasmal Tumors in Children

J. Lawton Smith, M.D.

Two tumors commonly involve the optic chiasm in children. These are craniopharyngiomas and optic gliomas. Radiotherapy has been accepted as helpful in the former in many clinics, but controversy exists at this time as to the best management of the latter. It is important for the radiotherapist to obtain an ophthalmological consultation for quantitative measurement of the visual acuity and the visual fields prior to beginning therapy. Quantitative perimetry is indicated at the following times in all cases of chiasmal tumors:

1. before the craniotomy
2. after the craniotomy
3. before radiotherapy
4. during the course of radiotherapy
5. after radiotherapy.

Granted the above, how often should the visual fields be checked during the actual course of radiation?

1. once a week for three weeks (twice a week if visual loss is severe)
2. every two weeks for the next six weeks
3. every month for the next six months
4. every three months for a year thereafter
5. every six months until stable
6. once a year thereafter
7. improvement often occurs six to eight months after therapy
8. fields should be repeated whenever symptoms recur.

The author believes that craniopharyngioma is best managed initially by surgical exploration, determination if the lesion is solid or cystic, excision if feasible, and biopsy and decompression otherwise. Tumor recurrences are less if postoperative radiation is given. The author advises radiation of all cases of craniopharyngioma postoperatively unless the surgeon is convinced that total excision was accomplished. This is a rarity, and the late visual results and recurrence rate of craniopharyngioma continue to be unhappy as a rule. The

J. Lawton Smith, M.D., *Professor of Ophthalmology, Professor of Neurosurgery, University of Miami School of Medicine, Miami, Florida.*

author believes that radiation therapy should be advised postoperatively in many more cases of craniopharyngioma than is commonly done at this time.

As stated above, controversy exists as to best management of optic glioma at this time. One cause for this is failure to differentiate between tumors confined to the optic nerve and those of the chiasm. Another problem relates to the histopathology of the lesion in question. The following involve the optic nerve or its vaginal sheath: astrocytoma, spongioblastoma, glioblastoma multiforme, hamartoma, meningioma, neurofibroma, arachnoidal hyperplasia, and fibromatosis.

From the clinical point of view, optic gliomas are usually seen in children, and 90% occur before age 20. They present with visual loss, proptosis, strabismus, optic atrophy, and often show cafe-au-lait spots, optic canal enlargement, and J-shaped sellas. Effort should be made to define whether the lesion is confined to one optic nerve, or whether the other eye is involved, as the latter indicts the chiasm. Conventional therapy has been surgery for glioma of the nerve, and radiotherapy for glioma of the chiasm.

Recent reports have emphasized conservatism in the management of these tumors. A plea is made for careful study and follow-up of these patients. Shunting operations for hydrocephalus may be life saving in some instances. Dramatic improvement has been seen following radiotherapy in some cases. Steroids may be worth trying. While the controversy has helped in requiring better evaluation of these patients, compassionate and careful therapy may well offer the patient more than repeated studies with no therapy.

Malignant Lymphoma — Hodgkin's Disease — Originating in the Thyroid Region of a Child

Mario M. Vuksanovic, M.D.

Introduction

The thyroid gland as initial locus of any kind of malignant lymphoma at any age, sex, or race is an extremely rare occurrence.[1,7,8,10] Most of the reports of malignant lymphomas occurring in the thyroid gland deal with varieties other than Hodgkin's disease. Shimkin and Sagerman reported 11 cases of thyroid lymphoma in adults. It is only natural that there should be a great deal of reluctance among the clinicians and the pathologists to accept the diagnosis of primary lymphoma starting in the thyroid gland. This is even more so if the thyroid gland is postulated to be the primary site of a lymphomatous process in adolescence and even more so of Hodgkin's variety. For the same reason, only an uncontroversial, categorical, and extremely well-documented case would be free of doubts as to the authenticity of such happening. The main argument against Hodgkin's occurring as a primary site in the thyroid would naturally be the possibility that the gland has only secondarily been affected by the disease which had started in the lymphoid tissue and nodes of the head and neck area. Primary lymphosarcoma of the thyroid of adults has been reported to be at times associated with other pathological entities, such as thyroiditis, goiter.[6,11] Woolner found that some of the patients with lymphoma in the thyroid gland have also had increased positive titers of thyroid antibodies comparable to those encountered in Hashimoto's disease. Some authors, such as Cox and Lindsay, have speculated that there is more than mere coincidence between lymphomatous processes and co-existing thyroiditis. Up to the moment of these writings, only 13 cases of Hodgkin's disease have been accepted in medical

Mario M. Vuksanovic, M.D., *Clinical Professor of Radiology, University of Miami School of Medicine; Director, Department of Radiation Oncology, Cedars of Lebanon Medical Center, Miami, Florida.*
*From the Department of Radiotherapy, Cedars of Lebanon Hospital, Miami, Florida.

151

literature as originating in the thyroid. The material has been assembled by Mikal and is shown with slight modification in Table 1.

The patients reported in the literature presenting with a lymphomatous process originating in the thyroid gland were elderly, with predominance of lymphocytic lymphoma. When accompanied with a goiter, there appeared to be a slight predominance among the females.[8] Tumor masses localized in the thyroid gland suspected to be of a neoplastic nature are surgically removed. The entire specimen is available for histopathological study and associations with the existing or coincidental pathological entities are confirmed. In Woolner's series, however, a group of these patients were not considered operable by virtue of fixation to the underlying structures and/or extension outside of the gland. In these instances, the lesions were biopsied and subsequently treated by irradiation. Most of these patients with extensive involvement of the gland and extension to the retrosternal region were dyspneic, while some of them had also dysphagia. Local lymph node involvement was found in 20 and in five instances there was a Hashimoto's thyroiditis associated with lymphomatous process (Woolner).

Malignant lymphoma in children comprises about 6% of all childhood cancer.[9] In the immense majority of these patients (90% in Butler's series) an initial sign is that of peripheral lymph node enlargement. Out of 43 children reported by this author, 19 had cervical adenopathy on the right side, 21 of this series had lymphadenopathy on the left side of the neck, and 3 patients presented with bilateral adenopathy. He made no reference to possible secondary involvement of the thyroid gland by the lymphoma. It might be of interest that the time interval between the onset of symptoms and signs and the histological verification of the disease had been extremely variable, being in a

TABLE 1. Hodgkin's Disease*
With Primary Manifested in the Thyroid Gland — All Cases Included

Authors	Year of Report	No. of Cases
Kramer, E.	1930	1
Presno, Y. & Bastiony, J. S.	1936	1
Sternberg, C.	1936	2
Cohen, M. & Moore, G. E.	1954	1
Rovello, F.	1955	3
Smithers, D. W.	1955	3
Roberts, T. W. & Howard, R. G.	1963	2**
Total		13

*Modified from Stanley Mikal.
**One case contributed by Meissner.

few patients as long as several months and even years duration. Seventy-seven children harbored Hodgkin's disease of a nodular sclerosing type. One of his patients presumably affected by generalized Hodgkin's disease had the tumor histologically verified in the soft tissues of the knee.

Material and Method

From 1962 through 1971, inclusive, the records of 13 selected infant patients with early (Stage I and II) histologically verified Hodgkin's disease were reviewed. This comprises a fraction of a total of 52 children seen with this diagnosis in the Division of Radiation Therapy at Jackson Memorial Hospital and the Department of Radiation Therapy at Cedars of Lebanon Hospital. The purpose was to ascertain the initial site of Hodgkin's disease.

Table 2 summarizes the distribution of these 13 cases with Hodgkin's lymphoma, according to sex, stage, and median age. Seven of these infants were males: three were Staged clinically I and four were Staged II. Among the six females, two were Staged I and four were affected by Stage II disease. No patient of this group underwent Staging laparotomy. Eleven had conventional bilateral pedal lymphangiography as part of their workup. All of the patients had chest plate IVP, peripheral blood count, bone marrow, and other usual laboratory studies (urine, etc.). Not a single case exhibited constitutional symptoms.

Table 3 summarizes the recorded anatomical regions of the initial clinical manifestation of the lymphoma. Six patients had cervical adenopathy on the left; three patients had a single manifestation on the right side of the neck; two patients presented with mediastinal widening only and the diagnosis was confirmed through exploratory thoracotomy. A single infant of this series had Hodgkin's disease predominantly in the thyroid region and is subsequently presented with some detail.

Figure 1 shows distribution of the anatomically compromised area by the disease in this selected group of children. As mentioned, a single youth when first seen presented with predominantly involved thyroid gland by the Hodgkin's

TABLE 2. Distribution of 13 Cases (Early)* with Hodgkin's Disease (Stage I-II) According to Sex, Stage, and Median Age

7 Males		6 Females	
Stage I	*Stage II*	*Stage I*	*Stage II*
3	4	2	4
Ages: Youngest 6 years; oldest 15 years; Median: 11 years.			

*None with constitutional symptoms at initial examination.

TABLE 3. Initial Clinical Manifestation in Stages I-II (Early)
Hodgkin's Disease in 13 Children

Cervical Lymph Nodes					
Left Nodes		Right Nodes			
Alone	*With Others**	*Alone*	*With Others*	*Mediastinum Alone (Thoracotomy)*	*Thyroid Alone*
3	3	3	1	2	1

*Bilateral nodes, axillae – single or both, mediastinum, etc.

disease. Considering the exceedingly extreme rarity in which the disease process has its onset in the thyroid gland, not only in infants but in the entire human population, it would be an extremely difficult if not impossible task to prove that this particular patient had the onset of his Hodgkin's lymphoma in the thyroid gland itself. On the other hand, the possibility of coincidental acute thyroiditis might be a more readily acceptable proposition.

Case Report, J.G.

A 13-year-old male was admitted to the Department of Pediatrics at Jackson Memorial Hospital, Miami, Florida, in early July, 1968, with a history of acute swelling of the neck, of two weeks duration. His past medical history was entirely unremarkable. Upon examination on July 4, 1968, he presented with respiratory difficulties and a non-productive cough. He was afebrile although acutely ill and dyspneic with inspiratory stridor. Pertinent physical findings were

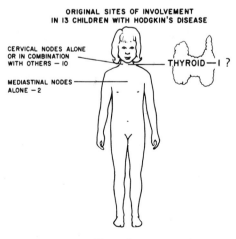

ORIGINAL SITES OF INVOLVEMENT
IN 13 CHILDREN WITH HODGKIN'S DISEASE

CERVICAL NODES ALONE
OR IN COMBINATION
WITH OTHERS – 10

THYROID—1 ?

MEDIASTINAL NODES
ALONE – 2

Figure 1.

that of thyroid enlargement, somewhat more prominent on the left side of the neck. It extended semicircumferentially, the entire tumefaction estimated to measure 12 × 8 cm in greatest diameter. The entire thyroid gland was replaced by a smooth, extremely tender, and firm in consistency almost woodened tumor mass. It extended from the thyroid cartilage downward towards the suprasternal notch. There was mention of questionable left supraclavicular fossa adenopathy on this initial examination. Roentgenogram of the chest at that time presented extension of the neck mass toward the anterior and superior mediastinal region. The trachea appeared narrowed and displaced towards the left side and posteriorly. This component of the tumor appeared extremely suggestive of substernal thyroid extension. The laboratory data were as follows: CBC and differential were within normal limits; BEI was 7.2; PBI 13.2; and Iodine-131 uptake at 24 hours was 8%. The remaining laboratory examinations were within normal limits. On July 26, he was started on prednisone with the initial dose of 40 mg daily. He was simultaneously given T_3, 75µg daily. The admitting diagnosis was that of acute thyroiditis. With this management, the child's symptoms appeared to improve somewhat. He was discharged from the hospital on July 31, 1968 to continue on 40 mg of prednisone daily. He was considered to be euthyroid at the time of discharge. The patient continued on prednisone and triiodothyronine on an outpatient basis. An attempt to decrease the daily prednisone to 20 mg resulted immediately in exacerbation of his symptomatology. The thyroid region remained enlarged, firm, and the initial tenderness, while decreased somewhat in intensity, had not disappeared. Due to the extent and fixation of the tumor mass in the neck, the medical management above described was considered as an alternative to surgery. Nevertheless, the pediatrician in charge became extremely doubtful of his initial diagnosis of acute thyroiditis alone. He commented that the persistence of tumefaction and tenderness could be attributed to massive subcapsular hemorrhage into the thyroid gland. He did not discard, however, the thyroiditis as concomitant process in view of the fact that there was symptomatic relief upon the administration of corticosteroids.

On October 15, 1968, an attempt was recorded to decrease the daily intake of prednisone to 20 mg daily, a circumstance which again resulted in exacerbation of his respiratory symptomatology. At this time the child was noted to present some Cushinoid characteristics while the thyroid mass remained essentially unchanged. There was no mention of the presence of peripheral adenopathy; however, the chest plate at that time demonstrated some improvement, a slight decrease of the substernal mass, and less compression of the trachea.

Finally, on December 12, 1968, the youth was referred to the Surgical Department, Harkness Pavilion – Presbyterian Hospital, New York City. The pediatric surgeon identified a small, left supraclavicular node and performed open biopsy of the mass. The patient still presented with persistent enlargement of the thyroid region and tenderness. The histological report rendered was that of Hodgkin's disease in the left supraclavicular node. He was referred back to Miami to the Department of Pediatrics, University of Miami School of Medicine, Jackson Memorial Hospital with the suggestion to offer the child a course of radiotherapy. He was then referred to the Division of Therapeutic Radiology at the same institution and from then on he was managed and followed in the Division of Radiotherapy with the diagnosis of Hodgkin's disease, Stage I without constitutional symptoms. The histopathological material was reviewed by the Department of Pathology at Jackson Memorial Hospital, University of Miami School of Medicine. Figures 2 and 3 are microphotographs representative of the specimen of the node procured from the left supraclavicular region.

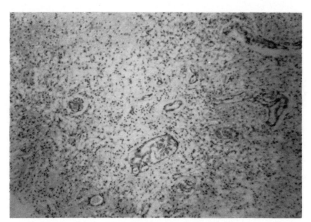

Figure 2.

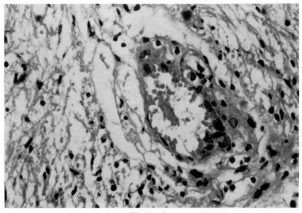

Figure 3.

Initial examination in Radiotherapy was done on July 24, 1968. Physical examination at this point disclosed a boy of normal development for his age. A large, anterior neck mass estimated at 12×10 cm in greatest diameter, occupying semicircumferentially the entire anterior neck from the thyroid cartilage down to the suprasternal notch, was again noticed. He was still dyspneic and Cushinoid in appearance. The neck tumefaction was uniformly smooth, slightly tender, and extremely firm in consistency. The remaining physical examination disclosed moderate hypertrophy of adenoid tissue in the oronasal pharynx. There were no other abnormalities or palpable adenopathy present. There were no abnormal abdominal masses or visceromegaly encountered. Figure 4 is the lateral and frontal view of the neck mass.

Figure 5 is a roentgenogram of the chest obtained on December 26, 1968. It confirmed the clinical diagnosis of enlarged neck mass with mediastinal widening. There was no calcification apparent within the mass, however.

Figure 6 is a left lateral view roentgenogram illustrating a large mass with its superior and anterior mediastinal component.

The subsequent figure demonstrates abdominal distention encountered on the initial examination of this 13-year-old boy, with distention of the subcutaneous tissues and striae, a consequence of hypercorticism iatrogenically induced (Fig. 7).

The clinical picture was misleading to the extent that the final diagnosis was delayed for several months, while the patient became Cushinoid by virtue of administration of corticosteroids. This iatrogenically induced syndrome was clearly apparent in this 13-year-old boy on his initial consultation visit at the Division of Radiation Therapy. The symptomatology resulting from the mechanical compression of the trachea by the large tumor mass persisted until such time that specific therapy (irradiation), was instituted following the establishment of the true disease process. The bilateral low-extremity lymphangiogram subsequently performed, liver scan, bone marrow, and excretory urogram were all within normal limits.

Therapy

The radiation therapy consisted of modification of the "upper mantle" that included lymph node bearing regions from the Waldayer's Ring to the mediastinum with the exclusion of the axillae. A 6 MEV Linear Accelerator at 100 cm focal skin distance was used. The portal of treatment thus included the entire neck, both supraclavicular fossae, and mediastinum. Irradiation began on January 2, 1969, ending on January 30, 1969. A minimum tumor dose estimated at a 10 cm depth from this single anterior perpendicular portal was that of 3300 rads. The estimated dose at 1 cm depth was that of 4550 rads. Lungs were shielded by shaped lead blocks 6 inches thick. The larynx was not protected so that at the end of treatment the patient presented moderate

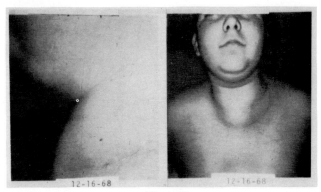

Figure 4.

dysphasia, hoarseness, and mild cutaneous reactions. He was gradually taken off prednisone and was placed on a high protein-low caloric diet. On follow-up examination of February 16, 1969, a residual tumor mass confined to the thyroid region was still present. A "booster dose" to this area was administered

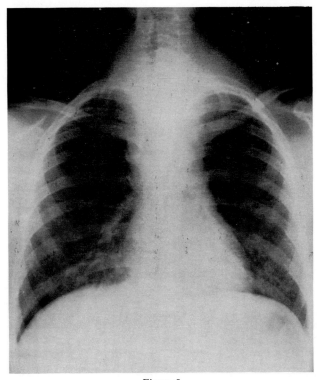

Figure 5.

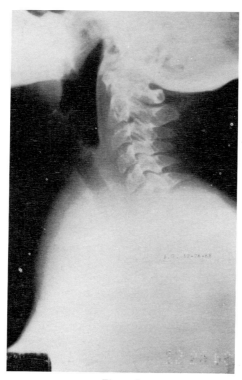

Figure 6.

with Cobalt 60 teletherapy unit, focal skin distance 80 cm and was given to an additional dose of 1000 rads estimated at a 2 cm depth in five consecutive treatments at increment doses of 200 rads. His second course of treatment ended on February 24, 1969. He was referred to an endocrinologist for evaluation of

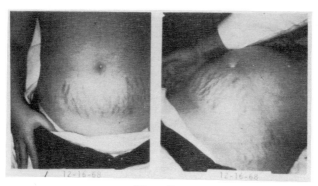

Figure 7.

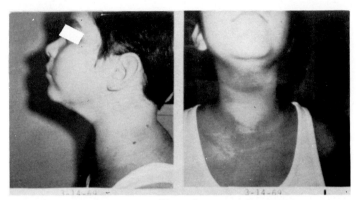

Figure 8.

his thyroid function. Some deficiency was expected to be encountered as a consequence of the alteration of the normal glandular tissue by replacement and scarring induced by the intensive radiation treatment. On the other hand the thyroid function tests were omitted because of the recent lymograms. He was given 2 gr of thyroid daily under close scrutiny by the endocrinologist.

On follow-up examination of March 4, 1969, the patient was found free of adenopathy in any area and his irradiation-induced symptomatology was no longer present. His voice was normal and he no longer complained of dysphasia. Thorough examination of the neck area failed to reveal tenderness or abnormalities. Figure 8 was obtained at this examination.

Subsequent follow-up studies showed complete disappearance of masses, both clinically and roentgenographically. This could be well appreciated in Figures 9 and 10 obtained on June 30, 1969 and November 15, 1971. The youth has continued normal in every respect, exhibiting no handicaps of a developmental nature. Figure 11 is a frontal view of the chest plate obtained on

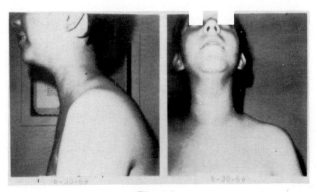

Figure 9.

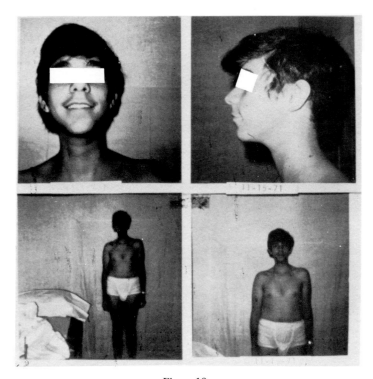

Figure 10.

November 15, 1971. He is currently being followed at regular intervals in the Department of Radiation Therapy at Cedars of Lebanon Hospital, Miami, Florida. The last examination done in December 1972 was uneventful; the patient remained free of clinical or roentgenological evidence of his Hodgkin's disease.

Discussion and Summary

Hodgkin's disease in childhood is extremely rare. Hodgkin's lymphoma originating in the thyroid gland as a single manifestation in infants or adolescents has not been authentically proven to the present time. It is not this author's intention whatsoever to report a 14th case of Hodgkin's disease originating in the human thyroid. Instead, a retrospective review of this case is extremely suggestive of a coincidental onset of Hodgkin's disease and a pathological process of the thyroid gland in a 13-year-old youth with an uneventful past medical history. This association of malignant lymphoma of Hodgkin's variety with pathological process of the thyroid gland is indeed extremely rare and in itself presents considerable medical interest. The relationship of enlargement of the

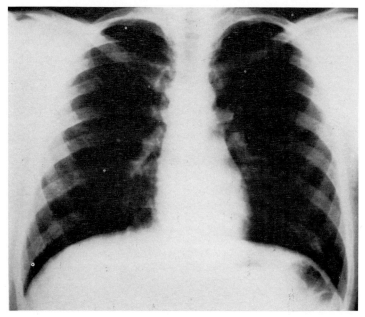

Figure 11.

thyroid gland in the neck with mediastinal widening could be interpreted as substernal component of the gland producing symptomatology confined to the upper respiratory passage. In fact it has misled an experienced pediatrician to the point of delaying the final diagnosis for several months. Thus initially, the clinical picture presented as acute thyroiditis. The primary locus of Hodgkin's lymphoma in the thyroid gland cannot be substantiated. The histological material was procured from the left supraclavicular node. Even though it may have represented at that point an extracapsular extension of the lymphoma in the thyroid, evidence is lacking that the thyroid was the site of Hodgkin's involvement since the glandular tissue itself was not examined. Nevertheless, the coincidence is such that speculation is at least a permissible proposition. The evidence at hand instead points out to the association of thyroiditis with Hodgkin's lymphoma.

References

1. Butler, J. J.: *Hodgkin's Disease in Children.* Chicago:Year Book Medical Publishers, 1969, pp. 267-279.
2. Cox, T. M.: Malignant lymphoma of the thyroid. *J. Clin. Path.* 17:591-601, 1964.
3. Crile, G., Jr.: Lymphosarcoma and reticulum cell sarcoma of the thyroid. *Surg. Gynec. Obstet.* 116:449-500, 1963.

4. Fujimoto, Y., Suzuki, H., Abe, K. and Brooks, R. J.: Autoantibodies in malignant lymphoma of the thyroid gland. *New Eng. J. Med.* 276:380-383, 1967.
5. Jenkin, R. D. T., Peters, M. V. and Darte, J. M. M.: Hodgkin's disease in children. *Amer. J. Roentgen.* 100:222-226, May, 1967.
6. Lindsay, S. and Dailey, M. E.: Malignant lymphoma of the thyroid gland and its relation to Hashimoto's disease – Clinical and pathological study of 8 patients. *J. Clin. Endocr.* 15:1332-1353, 1955.
7. Mikal, S.: Primary lymphoma of the thyroid gland. *Surgery* 55:233-239, 1964.
8. Pitcock, J. A., Bauer, W. C. and McGavran, M. H.: Hodgkin's disease in children: A clinicopathological study of 46 cases. *Cancer* 12:1043-1051, 1959.
9. Schneider, M.: Malignant lymphoma in children, in F. Buschke (ed): *Progress in Radiation Therapy.* New York:Grune & Stratton, 1965, vol 3, pp. 172-182.
10. Shimkin, M. P. and Sagerman, R. H.: Lymphoma of the thyroid gland. *Radiol.* 92:812-816, 1969.
11. Woolner, L. B., McConahey, M., Beahrs, H. O. and Black, M. B.: Primary malignant lymphoma of the thyroid – Review of 46 cases. *Amer. J. Surg.* 3:502-523, 1966.

Does Letterer - Siwe Disease Exist? Or, Who's Not Afraid of Infantile Histiocytes?

Gordon F. Vawter, M.D.

I am not sure that anything that I have to discuss with you has any direct therapeutic implications. However, we all believe that rational bases of therapy depend upon the degree of our understanding of the basic process with which we deal. Therapy in Letterer-Siwe disease will remain empiric for some time. There are, however, faint glimmerings that the millenium will come.

First, perhaps I should define Letterer-Siwe disease, for there has been a tendency in the recent past to consider all histiocytoses equivalent. My definition of Letterer-Siwe disease is: this is a characteristic histiocytosis. It has a clinical onset in infancy. (One may have a clinical onset before birth). The etiology is unknown and this requires exclusion of all identifiable causes. It is not leukemic. It is not truly granulomatous. And it is not familial. The points which will be discussed are some of the newer morphological concepts, some ideas about chemical aberrations which punctuate the process, and some comments on involvement of the thymus in Letterer-Siwe disease.

We are still, unfortunately, in the stage of descriptive morphology when we discuss Letterer-Siwe disease. The greatest advance which I can report to you, is still in the realm of descriptive morphology.

Dr. Christian Netzeloff and his group in Paris is responsible for the major advance in our understanding of the morphologic basis of Letterer-Siwe disease.[1] This advance consists of the demonstration of a characteristic intercellular body or granule resembling lesions by electron microscopic study of Letterer-Siwe the Langerhans granule. Figure 1 depicts the typical skin lesion of a Letterer-Siwe histiocytosis with an infiltrate of histiocytes hugging the epidermis and admixed with the epideral cells, recapitulating, perhaps, the normal distribution of Langerhans histiocytes.

The characteristic Langerhans body or granule is seen in Figure 2. It is a 5-layered membrane with central periodicity which has continuity with the

Gordon F. Vawter, M.D., *Associate Professor of Pathology, Children's Hospital Medical Center, Harvard Medical School, and Associate Pathologist-in-Chief of The Children's Hospital Medical Center, Boston, Mass.*

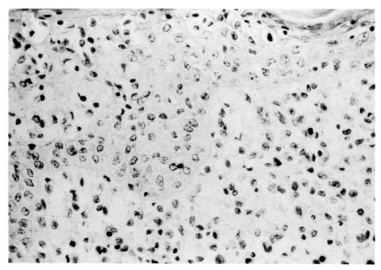

Fig. 1. Epidermis (top 1/3) and superficial dermis are infiltrated, predominantly by histiocytic cells with pale, oval or folded nuclei. H&E stain.

surface of the cell and with intracytoplasmic vesicles: its function is unknown. It is, however, a normal component of the dendritic histiocytes of the squamous epithelium first described by Langerhans; hence, the name of the granule. These structures which connect the surface of the cell with vesicles in the cytoplasm have been studied by others in terms of permeability. What we know from their work is that the granules are permeable to small ions but not to small protein molecules.[2] However, the cells which bear these granules contain lytic enzymes such as esterase, acid phosatase and peptidases which we expect in histiocytes. Whether these cells have immunologic function is unknown. Recently, at a meeting in Toronto,* Dr. Netzeloff reported his experience in studying histiocytoses by electron microscope. He reported 65 cases; 20 of these cases were Letterer-Siwe disease, and cells with this characteristic morphology were found in all. Interestingly enough, he found that in 15 cases of Hand-Schuller-Christian disease and in the remaining cases which represented eosinophilic granuloma of the lung, cells with this characteristic granule were present in all lesions. This tells us that the suspicions of a morphologic similarity or identity between these three clinically disparate groups, is, in fact, true. Dr. Netzeloff work in Columbus, Ohio, and less extensive work in our own laboratory, has clearly demonstrated that not all histiocytoses contain these recognizable Langerhans-like granules. It is on this morphologic basis that we may begin to wonder whether we cannot separate what is truly a Letterer-Siwe type histiocytosis from others?

---

*Pediatric Pathology Club, November, 1971, Hospital for Sick Children of Toronto.

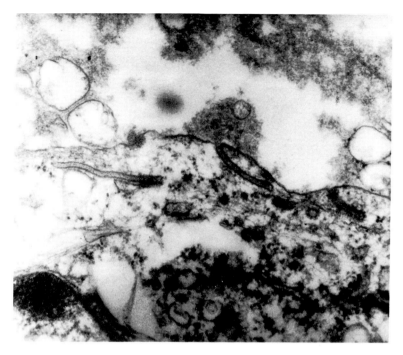

Fig. 2. Electron-micrograph of histiocytic containing Langerhans-like bodies (5 layered with central periodicity), 2 of which come to cell surface (courtesy of Dr. Betty Uzman, Division of Ultrastructural Research, Children's Cancer Research Foundation, Boston).

Netzeloff has advanced the hypothesis that Letterer-Siwe disease then may well represent, a spread or systematization of the Langerhans cells to many sites. We don't know, however, where the Langerhans cell actually arises. We only know that it is normally found in squamous epithelium and in thymus. We know nothing of what actually controls its migration or localization.

I am going to tread on areas which I should perhaps leave to experts but it is my opinion that histiocytes are not particularly radiosensitive as compared to lymphocytes. We know, moreover, that the lesions of Letterer-Siwe disease are within reason exquisitely radiosensitive, taken singly. This raises the question of whether or not these granules of unknown function and origin may represent a marker for some peculiar mechanism of radiosensitivity which we don't understand. Alternatively, we could consider that radiation control of other cell populations besides this histiocyte may be the determinant of the reactions which you observe in your therapy.

Next I would like to comment upon the lipid and cholesterol storage, which punctuates the course of some patients with Letterer-Siwe disease. It has been long felt that the large size and the increasing duration of the lesion promote the accumulation of the lipid in the histiocytes in question. Modern chemistry has raised other questions of possible relationship. First, the cells which do accumulate cholesterol during the course of diseases such as Letterer-Siwe disease occur at sites which we know now to be very active in sterol metabolism. Notable examples are the skin and the liver. A new parameter of the cholesterol storage question may then be raised by the recognition in Letterer-Siwe disease of a subgroup in which obstructive jaundice apparently directly related to biliary involvement may be defined. However, it seems likely, thinking along the lines of the model of primary biliary cirrhosis that there may be recognizable alterations of cholesterol metabolism long before the patient becomes subject to obstructive jaundice.

In our clinical experience, obstructive Letterer-Siwe lesions in the liver have been a grave prognostic sign. Another prospective area of valuable study of the cholesterol problem in Letterer-Siwe disease concerns the nature of the Langerhans granule. Sixty-percent of the cholesterol in cells is found in cell membranes. It is quite clear that the Langerhans granule is a cell membrane phenomenon.

One of the advances which gives some hope for defining the functional aspects of Letterer-Siwe disease rather than its infiltrative aspects is the advent of new methods of study. We have, together with Dr. George Foley's group at the Children's Cancer Research Foundation, established long term tissue culture of cells obtained from a patient with Letterer-Siwe disease. Such studies are also in progress in Japan, and in Paris. Only beginnings, however, have been made.

It is interesting to note that one can occasionally still find the Langerhans granule in these cells even after months of tissue culture. We have another form of histiocytosis in long term cell culture. We envisage rich opportunities to study and compare the function of these differing cell lines.

The next subject I would like to discuss is the relationship of the immunologic status of the host with Letterer-Siwe disease to the problems which we don't understand in these patients. First we should point out that symptomatic histiocytoses are prominent in well-defined states, such as hypogammaglobulinemia or in certain lymphopenias. But the fragmentary studies we have done in our own laboratories have failed so far to demonstrate Langerhans granules in this type of histiocytosis. Good has recently described Langerhans cells in the epidermal lesions which commonly complicate certain rare syndromes of granulocyte incompetence. Langerhans granules have also been described occasionally in other forms of histiocytosis, where cutaneous involvement is not rare. We need, therefore, to study all parameters of body defense in patients with Letterer-Siwe disease. Any cell which one can get in one's hand, I believe, is fit subject for intensive study in these patients. When Letterer first described this aleukemic reticulosis in 1924, he noted that the thymus was large, bright yellow, and greasy at autopsy. Since that time, when the thymus has been studied in patients with Letterer-Siwe disease, it has been consistently abnormal. In fact, in the past five years or so in our laboratory, thymic involvement by Letterer-Siwe histiocytosis has become one of the *sina qua non*'s of the diagnosis.

Essential features are those of a thymic histiocytosis which progresses to virtual destruction of the gland (Fig. 3). It seems likely, on morphologic grounds therefore, that thymic lymphocyte deficiency occurs at least late in Letterer-Siwe disease. It is now imperative that we study the parameters of thymic function as early as possible in the patient with Letterer-Siwe disease and serially after the diagnosis, for it may be that one point-of-no-return in Letterer-Siwe disease, as compared with the other syndromes where Langerhans histiocytes are involved, may revolve around this effect of destruction of the thymic gland.

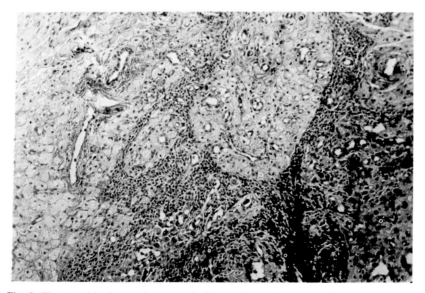

Fig. 3. The atrophic thymus is surrounded by and contains groups of histiocytes. H&E stain.

Early in Letterer-Siwe disease, there is morphologic evidence of adequate lymphoid follicular activity, whereas even early, there may be morphologic deficiency of areas associated with thymic lymphocytes.

In summary, we have discussed briefly the possible significance of the Langerhans histiocyte; intercurrent biochemical abnormalities of Letterer-Siwe disease; and finally, the role that the thymus may play in the course of Letterer-Siwe disease.

References

1. Basset, et al.: *Comptr Rendar Acad. Sci.* (Paris) 261:3701, 1965.
2. Hashimoto, K.: Lanthanum Staining of Langerhans Cells, *Arch. Derm.* 102:280, 1970.

Supportive Care of Patients with Malignant Disease

C. Dean Buckner

Supportive care of patients with malignant disease is a sufficiently broad topic to enable me to discuss a variety of subjects. I would like to discuss today some of the progress that has been made in the area of cellular supportive measures in patients with marrow failure, specifically platelet and granulocyte transfusions. If time permits, I may also make a few comments about marrow infusions and ultraisolation techniques. Most of the topics I will discuss today are investigative in nature and not in general use; however, I hope some of my comments may relate to some of the problems encountered in the management of pediatric patients with malignancy.

Dr. Burchenal discussed the importance of intensive early treatment of leukemia and emphasized the survivors. The content of much of the work I will discuss pertains more to the non-responders and those that are refractory to treatment which, unfortunately, is still the majority of patients with malignant disease, especially in the adult.

One of the reasons I have chosen to emphasize the supportive care of marrow failure is the magnitude of the problem. The chemotherapeutic agents and irradiation we use produce pancytopenia and immunosuppression with resultant hemorrhage and infection. Hemorrhage and infection account for 98% of deaths in patients with leukemia.[1] This reflects the end results of the basic disease process plus the results of treatment with cytotoxic agents. The basic problem remains to improve the methods of treatment of the underlying disease state. However, at the present time, we have to use the agents that are available and cope with the complications of infection and hemorrhage.

Hemorrhage, in most patients with malignancy, is due to thrombocytopenia, although this is often more complicated than a simple production defect. The incidence of hemorrhage is related to the absolute level of platelets and the number of days spent at low levels as has been pointed out by Dr. Freireich and

C. Dean Buckner, *Department of Medicine, University of Washington School of Medicine, Seattle, Washington and the U.S. Public Health Service Hospital, Seattle, Washington.*

This work is supported by grants CA 10895, CA 10167 and CA 12190 and contract AI 09419 from the National Institutes of Health, U.S. Public Health Service.

his colleagues several years ago.[1] This propensity for bleeding can also be measured by bleeding times. In our laboratory the normal bleeding time done on the forearm with a standardized cut is 4½ minutes. Dr. Slichter, in our division, has correlated the bleeding time with the platelet level and shown a steady increase in bleeding time beginning at platelet levels of 100,000 per mm[3]. At levels of 20,000 per mm[3] the bleeding time loses its sensitivity, which is unfortunate, as this is the range where we would most like to have a predictive test for bleeding. Dr. Slichter's studies in patients with aplastic anemia have demonstrated no loss of red cells in the stool at levels of 10,000 per mm[3] even though the bleeding time is over 60 minutes.[2]

For practical purposes we administer platelets to patients who have levels between 10 and 20,000 per mm[3] or to those who have bleeding even if their counts are higher. Using these criteria, we encounter very little in the way of clinical bleeding until immunization occurs. Patients who have a relatively intact immune system, as in aplastic anemia, will develop platelet refractoriness due to immunization very rapidly, while those on immunosuppressive chemotherapy tend to have a more delayed onset.

Platelet consumption is a common problem in malignancy and most, if not all, patients will have shortened platelet and fibrinogen survivals. Patients with sepsis have platelet and fibrinogen survivals of less than one day. The reason I emphasize these factors is that patients with severe thrombocytopenia with associated malignancy and infection need frequent platelet transfusions to keep them from bleeding. Often this will have to be done daily. The platelet consumption associated with malignancy will only get better with a remission in the disease and is not affected by heparin or coumarin.[2]

One can often get an idea of which mechanism is predominant, isoimmunization or consumption, by doing a 15 minute to 1 hour post-transfusion platelet count. Patients who are destroying platelets due to antibody usually do not have detectable increments, whereas patients with platelet consumption have a normal increment and a shortened platelet survival. Both mechanisms result in the same 24 hour post-transfusion platelet counts.

Therapeutically, we administer platelets to patients who have a consumptive process but not to those who have platelet antibodies. There is no definite proof that platelet transfusions are of value when the survival is less than 24 hours due to infection or malignancy, but my clinical impression is that they do. In the face of platelet refractoriness due to platelet isoimmunizations, the only maneuver that has been successful to date is platelet transfusions from histocompatible siblings. Transplantation antigens are carried on lymphocytes, granulocytes and platelets and can be utilized to type platelet donors and to detect sensitization. The major histocompatibility locus is located on a pair of autosomal chromosomes. With appropriate antisera, utilizing the lymphocytotoxicity test, it is possible to identify siblings who have inherited the same pair of parental autosomes carrying the histocompatibility locus. The lymphocytotoxicity test will also detect preformed antibodies in the recipient and although it is not as specific as other tests, it can be helpful in differentiating the etiology of platelet refractoriness.

Dr. Grumet and coworkers at the National Cancer Institute studied patients with aplastic anemia who were refractory to platelet transfusions from random donors.[3] Their patients had cytotoxic antibodies against 95% of random cells and against mismatched siblings. Platelets from random donors or mismatched siblings failed to elevate the platelet count, whereas, platelets from matched siblings survived normally. Two of these patients have been transfused for over a year and still respond normally to platelets from their matched HA-A siblings.

Typing of random donors for platelet transfusions has been generally unrewarding. A few phenotypically identical donor and recipient combinations have been tried without success. Occasionally, we have been able to use selected donors with negative crossmatches for short periods of time. We had a recent patient that was more typical, however. A 41-year-old multiparous female was admitted three weeks ago with acute leukemia and a platelet count of 9,000 per mm^3. She was transfused with platelets from random donors for two weeks and then became refractory. Cytotoxic antibodies were present against 70% of random donors. We selected a random donor who was antigenically similar, and to whom she did not have antibodies. The pre- and post-transfusion platelet counts were 3,000 per mm^3. Four units of platelets from her matched sibling, however, increased her platelet count to 60,000 per mm^3 with a three day survival.

Before I leave the subject of platelet transfusions, I would briefly like to mention two points for those interested in starting transfusion programs. Appropriate studies should be performed to assure the maximum platelet yield from a unit of blood and autologous *in vivo* platelet recoveries and survivals should be performed to assure platelet viability. Finally, platelets can be stored at room temperature for up to 72 hours.[4] This technique allows the clinician to have platelets available at night and on weekends as part of routine blood bank service.

I would like to now turn to the problem of granulocyte replacement. The relationship between granulocytopenia and infection is well known.[5] This, as with platelets, is a time versus level relationship. The longer the time spent at low granulocyte levels the greater the chance of infection. In contrast to red blood cells and platelets the granulocyte is difficult to replace. It makes up a small fraction of whole blood, survives in the blood for only a short period of time and is very fragile when manipulated. An average adult will produce and turn over 1×10^{11} granulocytes per day and several-fold this quantity under the stress of infection. Several years ago Dr. Freireich began transfusing granulocytes from donors with chronic myelogenous leukemia (CML) and, from his studies, he concluded that you needed 1×10^{11} granulocytes per meter of body surface area for predictable increments and therapeutic effectiveness.[6] Granulocytes from CML donors have one advantage over normal cells, they survive longer, presumably due to the maturing of immature cells in the recipient. These cells migrate to areas of infection and ingest bacteria in the recipient.[7] CML cells are satisfactory for transfusion but it is a relatively rare disease and donors are not usually available when you need them.

Granulocyte transfusions from normal donors have been difficult to evaluate. Utilizing the NCI-IBM blood cell separator, we can obtain 10×10^9 granulocytes from an adult in a four-hour period. This is obviously a small dose in comparison to the granulocyte turnover rate in the adult. Transfusion of this quantity into an adult rarely produces detectable increments. However, in a child, one can see granulocyte increments and survival. Granulocyte transfusions follow the same laws as platelets as far as immunization is concerned. In the presence of leukoaggluting or cytotoxic antibodies patients develop high fever, shaking chills and occasionally pulmonary infiltrates with respiratory insufficiency. Isoimmunization severely limits the usefulness of granulocyte transfusions, as it is a very frequent phenomena in patients who have received multiple blood transfusions.[7] Our studies in normal donors are, therefore, limited to recipients who do not have preformed antibodies.

Because of the relatively low numbers of granulocytes collected, and the rapid granulocyte turnover rate in the recipient, frequent transfusions are more logical. Dr. Graw at the National Cancer Institute had demonstrated that daily granulocyte transfusions are necessary to change the fatality rate from documented sepsis.[8]

The situation in which we utilize granulocytes is shown in the following case: A 13-year-old boy developed aplastic anemia associated with hepatitis. He was transferred to our research unit when he was discovered to have a HL-A matched sibling. At the time of admission he had a granulocyte count of 100 per mm^3 and a platelet count of 5,000 per mm^3. He was on amphotericin for a candida septicemia and admission cultures were still positive. We were fortunate to have a donor with CML available whose white blood cell count was 70,000 per mm^3 and who was ABO compatible. On alternate days the patient received granulocytes from the donor with CML obtained by multiple unit leukophoresis which amounted to between 40 and 90 billion granulocytes. On alternate days he received 10 to 20 billion granulocytes from his father collected with the NCI-IBM blood cell separator. Concomitant with this, he was pretreated with Cytoxan (CY) 200 mg/kg followed by a marrow graft from his HL-A matched sister. Transfusions maintained his granulocyte count during most of a three-week interval above 500 per mm^3 and frequently above 1,000 per mm^3. He cleared his infection and obtained a successful marrow transplant and is doing well four months later. It should be noted that at 21 days following engraftment, he developed cytotoxic antibodies against the CML donor but not his father.[9]

The overall question of the efficacy of granulocyte transfusions remains to be solved. There are many theoretical and some experimental reasons to believe that granulocyte transfusions under appropriate conditions will be beneficial. At the present time, however, we are still trying to obtain enough granulocytes to evaluate function and survival in a recipient and this work still remains very much in the realm of clinical research.

Summary

Two major problems in the supportive care of patients with malignant disease are hemorrhage and infection. Platelet transfusions have decreased the incidence of thrombocytopenic bleeding. However, transfusion therapy is frequently limited by platelet consumption due to underlying malignancy and infection and to isoimmunization. Frequent platelet transfusions and vigorous treatment of malignancy and infection are necessary to prevent bleeding. Platelets are of no value in the face of isoimmunization. Platelets from HL-A matched siblings will survive in situations where refractoriness exists to all other donors, and can be utilized when such a situation exists. The role of granulocyte replacement remains to be defined. This modality is subject to all the problems of platelet transfusions but is accentuated by the difficulty of procurement and the much shorter survival of granulocytes. Granulocytes from donors with chronic myelogenous leukemia are of value but donor availability is unpredictable. We are still working on improving the methods of procuring normal granulocytes for transfusion purposes. At the present time, the NCI-IBM continuous flow centrifuge is the best method available. There is some evidence that transfused normal granulocytes are beneficial but much work remains in this area to more precisely define their usefulness.

References

1. Hersh, E. M., Bodey, G. P., Nies, B. A., Freireich, E. J.: Causes of death in acute leukemia: A ten year study of 414 patients from 1954-1963. *JAMA* 193:105, 1965.
2. Slichter, S.: Unpublished observations.
3. Yankee, R. A., Grumet, F. C., and Rogentine, G. N.: Platelet transfusion therapy. The selection of compatible platelet donors for refractory patients by lymphocyte HL-A typing. *New Eng. J. Med.* 281:1208, 1969.
4. Murphy, S., Sayor, S. N., and Gardner, F. H.: Storage of plaetlet concentrates at 22°C. *Blood* 35:549, 1970.
5. Bodey, P., Buckley, M., Sathe, Y. S., and Freireich, E. J.: Quantitative relationship between circulating leukocytes and infection in patients with acute leukemia. *Ann. Int. Med.* 64:328, 1966.

6. Freireich, E. J., Levin, R. H., Whang, J., Carbone, P. P., Bronson, W., and Morse, E. E.: The function and fate of transfused leukocytes from donors with chronic myelocytic leukemia in leukopenic recipients. *Amer. N. Y. Acad. Sci.* 113:1081, 1964.
7. Eyre, H. J., Goldstein, I. M., Perry, S. and Graw, R. G.: Leukocyte transfusion: Function of transfused granulocytes from donors with chronic myelocytic leukemia. *Blood* 36:432, 1970.
8. Graw, R., Jr.: Unpublished observations.
9. Thomas, E. D., Buckner, C. D., Storb, R., Neiman, P. E., Fefer, A., Clift, R. A., Slichter, S. J., Funk, D. D., Bryant, J. I., and Lerner, K. E.: Aplastic anemia treated by marrow transplantation.

Psychological Issues in Caring for the Fatally Ill Child

Stanford B. Friedman, M.D.

Today I would like to share with you some of our observations regarding the psychological problems of fatally ill children and their parents, and to relate these findings to the views of others. In the way of introductory remarks, it should be realized that most of this information has been obtained from parents of children with leukemia. The natural course of this disease is rapidly changing, and there are few studies of psychological factors that have been made since childhood leukemia has had a more chronic course. Also, there is a real need for studies that would examine the psychological implications of physical problems such as cystic fibrosis and chronic kidney disease treated by renal transplantation.

Our own work has primarily focused on psychological coping mechanisms. I will concentrate on those areas that parents repeatedly bring up regarding caring for a fatally ill child, because of their immediate clinical application. Some of these points are rather simplistic, but the fact that parents repeatedly make these points means that our knowledge of the psychological implications of fatal illness is not always applied.

I would like to start my discussion at the point prior to the diagnosis, and then progress in chronological order. I start *before* the diagnosis as I believe we often underestimate the general public's medical sophistication regarding diseases such as cancer. Much of this is due, I am sure, to the lay press and also to the information given to the public related to fund-raising. What this means is that many parents are aware of the diagnostic possibilities even before they are mentioned to them. Prior to confirmation of the diagnosis the physician often avoids the topic of what the child may have. We, as physicians, do not wish to add stress to the situation for parents, and therefore do not like to share with them all of diagnostic possibilities, particularly those that have a fatal outcome. The physician should not raise the diagnostic possibility of neoplastic disease with the parents prior to the definitive diagnosis, but he should *allow* the question to emerge if the parents wish to raise it. This means that the physician

Stanford B. Friedman, M.D., *Departments of Pediatrics and Psychiatry, University of Rochester School of Medicine and Dentistry, Rochester, New York.*

177

has to provide sufficient time and privacy so that the parents have the opportunity to ask, "Do you think it might be cancer?" If the physician does not allow this opportunity, the doctor-patient relationship begins with an initial problem of communication. And, indeed, in retrospect, parents have recognized anger directed at physicians who did not allow them this expression of fear of the diagnosis.

Once the definitive diagnosis has been made, parents describe a feeling of "shock," "disbelief," or "unreality." This feeling of disbelief is not primarily intellectual denial." In other words, the parents intellectually accept the diagnosis but do not fully experience the emotional impact. What seems to be occurring is that severe psychological stresses have to be dealt with in a step-wise fashion. It is the organism's protection against becoming psychologically overwhelmed. The process of "emotional acceptance" may take days or even weeks. This should not be viewed in the same light as complete intellectual denial of the diagnosis which may interfere with medical care. All of you are aware of occurrences of this sort, where the parents will not allow the diagnostic procedure or therapy to continue because they deny at all levels the fact that their child has a neoplastic disease. These are the parents who will often go to multiple medical facilities or worse, from our viewpoint, seek out inappropriate medical or non-medical help.

It is usual for the husband to support his wife early in the course of their child's illness. For the first few days, the father typically makes the important family decisions, allowing his wife to experience more emotion than he does. The husband may truly "Feel" the impact of the diagnosis only some days or weeks following the time when his wife no longer needs such intensive support. One reason for emphasizing this point is that in cases of divorce or death, the remaining parent has an especially difficult time adapting as there is no opportunity for mutual support.

The implications for the physician from this are, I believe, several. First, in talking about the diagnosis, there is a need for privacy. I think that all of us would acknowledge this and yet parents are still told about the diagnosis in the hallways and in the presence of other individuals. Sitting down with the parents, rather than standing, promotes a feeling in parents that the physician is not eager to leave as soon as possible.

Second, early after the parents learn of the diagnosis, explanations to the patients and parents should be kept simple. Parents often tell us that they did not understand the medical language or the complexity of the medical situation. What they want is primarily the information needed to comprehend, in a general way, the situation, so as to understand the recommendations of the physician. The physician should plan to convey the more detailed explanation of the illness by a series of discussions rather than try to explain everything all at once. There is a need for repeated explanations which follows from varying degrees of denial of the diagnosis. The parents in essence are asking over and over again – some more than others – "Does my child really have this disease?" Part of the process of acceptance of the diagnosis is to hear the doctor state it repeatedly, and this does not mean that the parents are mentally dull or have psychiatric problems.

I would now like to introduce the concept of anticipatory guidance, in that parents can be forewarned that certain things are likely to happen, and if they are forewarned they are better able to cope with them. For instance, friends and family often represent added stress to parents. Relatives, particularly, often make statements such as "Johnny can't have leukemia as he looks too healthy." They will send newspaper and magazine articles which often *appear* to contradict what the physician has said, or introduce unrealistic hope into the situation. In other words, the friends and relatives tend to support denial of the disease. They try to introduce hope but in reality it is a false kind of hope. One mother put this very well when she said, "It is as if I am the only one who believes that my son has leukemia and I have to keep telling others that he has it. It is beginning to get so that I almost feel as if I am *giving him* leukemia."

At the same time that friends and relatives support the denial of the disease, they paradoxically often do not allow parents to even partially return to previous modes of living. For instance, a mother of a child who has been treated for leukemia for about one year, gave a birthday party for one of her other children. She promptly received a letter from her mother condemning her for this, which said "How can you give a birthday party when one of your children is dying?" This same grandmother had been sending newspaper clippings about "cures" and suggesting that the diagnosis of leukemia might in itself be wrong. Thus, relatives frequently foster denial of the disease, yet make it difficult for parents to partially return to their usual life style and activities.

When the child is hospitalized, the mother generally is more comfortable caring for him than is the father. She has a role that is not too dissimilar from her previous role as a mother. Fathers are, as one father put it, "all thumbs." Because of this, and for other reasons, fathers may spend significantly less time on the ward, and do not have continuing contact with the physician. This puts the mother in the difficult role, in a sense, of translating the doctor's communications to the father, who may then ask "What did he mean by that?" The mother then must return to the physician to ask him the questions asked by the father of her. This often causes unnecessary anxiety and sometimes conflict between the parents that would be eliminated if communications were directed to both of them.

It is rare for physicians to discuss with parents what the siblings should be told, and yet parents frequently need help in this area. What and how to tell siblings must, of course, take into account their ages and other developmental considerations. An extreme case illustrates the fact that siblings are often ignored in the total management of families having a fatally ill child:

I was asked to see the parents of a child who was terminally ill with leukemia as their two teenage daughters had been repeatedly told their brother had some sort of anemia and apparently were not aware of the seriousness of his illness. The house officer was appropriately concerned as to how they would react to his death. The girls had never been allowed to visit their brother in the hospital, and the parents were now concerned as to what to say to their daughters and asked me to talk to them. This I agreed to do, but the boy died during the night. The parents were left not only with their grief over his death, but also the problem of how belatedly to deal honestly with their two teenage daughters.

As the terminal phase of the disease approaches, anticipatory grief is noted in the majority of parents. This process includes the parents partially "deinvesting" themselves from the ill child, and the return of previous interests and activities. One mother put it this way: "I still love my boy every bit as much, but I feel less involved. I feel more detached." Another mother began to pack up her child's toys in anticipation of the fact that he would no longer be needing them. In this latter case, a nurse responded: "What are you doing? You are giving up hope! The doctors are still treating your child. *They* are still trying.' The mother was, in effect, reprimanded for going through the anticipatory grieving process.

Parents also show anticipatory grief by turning their attention to other children. Their own child may be very seriously ill, but we find the parents may pay more attention to other children, even children who are in the hospital for some minor problem. Again, if allowed to be expressed, one will almost always see this kind of grieving before the actual death of the child. When such expression of grieving is not allowed to occur, the death itself may be accepted in a totally different way by parents. Typically, parents will describe death following a long illness as the "last step down" or the "final event" if anticipatory grieving has occurred. If this has not occurred, parents have more difficulty coping with the death of their child in that grieving begins more acutely. And, indeed, some parents are unable to resolve the loss even after the death. The continuing denial of the loss and the inability to grieve may lead to abnormal behavior, that though not common, usually warrants psychiatric intervention. An example were young parents who lost their only child, a 2-year-old son with leukemia. Rather than try to conceive another child of their own, they adopted another boy of the same age in an inappropriate attempt to replace the dead child.

During the terminal phase of a child's illness, parents will often become preoccupied with laboratory results and details regarding medical management. What we are seeing here is an attempt by the parents to dwell upon the least threatening aspects of the disease. It is less threatening for many parents to psychologically cope with fluctuating white counts than with the fact that their child is terminal. Physicians often encourage this process to the point where the parents are, in effect, part of the therapeutic team. Parents will sometimes talk about this as being "in on" the medical decisions that are being made. They are in a sense being encouraged to think about the details of medical management, and not being helped in facing the problem that their child is dying.

It should be obvious that the parents should not participate in making medical decisions, particularly those related to the nature of the terminal therapy. If the child's life is prolonged by such therapy, they may experience guilt in that they have prolonged the suffering. On the other hand, if the child's life is not prolonged, they feel guilty about not having encouraged the physician to continue treatment.

I would now like to discuss the child himself. First, the conceptualization of death is age-dependent. In general, a child younger than 7 or 8 years of age perceives death as a reversible phenomenon or analogous to sleep. His fears are that of being abandoned and of experiencing pain.* As he progresses in age to the early teens, his thinking about death is more like that of the adult and his main fear may be of dying.

The fear that young children have of being abandoned has not been given enough attention. For instance, radiation services are for the most part designed for adults and not for children. Children are often left, at least as seen by the children, for long periods of time in hallways, frequently with very sick adults being wheeled past them. This type of abandonment is a very frightening experience for children.

The youngster is often confused about his illness. When he previously had, as an example, a sore throat, his illness was explained and his discomfort acknowledged. Contrast this to his now having a fatal disease. Often little is discussed with him about his illness and his pain and discomfort denied. He may be on the hospital ward with IV's running and nasal packs in, and yet everyone seems relatively cheerful and unconcerned. On morning rounds, the doctors come in and say, "You look fine today." This obviously conflicts with how he feels, and the child is confused and frightened. Frightened because "If the doctors think I am fine (or if my parents think I am fine), how are they ever going to help me?" This lack of understanding leads a search for non-verbal cues from the environment in an attempt to define what adults really think about his condition. There also may be overt "testing" as in the case of one 17-year-old boy. He asked his doctor, "What did my last bone marrow show?" The doctor told him of the findings. Then the boy, when the physician wasn't in the room, asked his mother and then his father, the same question. He then openly challenged them: "Each of you is telling me a different thing and I don't believe any of you." This is not to say that one spends the majority of time with the child in talking about his illness or in commiserating with him, but both

---

*There is, at times, an unnecessary reluctance of physicians to prescribe adequate medication for pain. This, of course, results in added distress, both physical and psychologic, for the child.

physicians and parents should acknowledge his concerns and feelings. Only then will cheerful talk and play be most effective.

Out of the hospital, a fatal illness often leads to overprotection, over-indulgence, and social isolation of the child. Parents may not allow their child to return to school or live a normal life even when the child feels well, as they fear he will hear that he has leukemia or cancer from friends. Physicians often tell parents what the child cannot do, but rarely emphasize what the child *can do* upon discharge from the hospital. Further, the parents may extend our restrictions and the child becomes essentially isolated from his friends and kept from participating in activities that are not medically contraindicated.

Hospitalization itself does not have to be all or nothing, and the child may be allowed to have "passes." I believe that all too often a child is kept in the hospital over a weekend for procedures which are to take place on Monday, and that he could have spent this time at the zoo or at home. In short, there is no reason, in many cases, for the child to have to stay in the hospital on a 24-hour basis. The latter is often for the convenience of hospital staff, not for the child.

There remains the difficult question of what to "tell" the child. First, as with the parents, the child should have an opportunity to ask questions. Morning work rounds are not the proper setting for such a discussion. Rather, the physician must be able to sit down for at least a few minutes and allow questions to emerge. Often this is not done as there is the fear that the child will ask, "Am I going to die?" It would appear that this question is rarely raised by children. They are more apt to ask, "Do I have a blood disease?" and then go on to ask "Do I have a low cell count?" or "Is my blood thin?" Even if the child asks if he has leukemia, he can be encouraged to rephrase the question, which often will reflect his quest for some information about the type of disease he has rather than whether it is fatal.

In an article entitled "Who is Afraid of Death on a Leukemia Ward?" Vernick and Karon forcefully raised the issue of what children should be told regarding their disease. They believe that older children should be told their diagnosis and argue that this practice protects the child from social isolation. There should, however, be some guidelines for this, and the foremost is to talk to a child about his diagnosis when he has already experienced some degree of therapeutic success, either through surgery or chemotherapy.

Summary

Fatal illness in childhood requires psychological adaptation on the part of the child, parents and siblings. An understanding by the physician of the frequent modes of psychological and social functioning of all family members is necessary for the optimal medical management of the fatally ill child. The physicians caring for children with fatal diseases should see the family as the "patient," realizing that parents and siblings of the ill child can also benefit from his skills and support.

Acknowledgement

The author wishes to acknowledge support from U. S. Public Health Grant K3-MH-18,542, awarded by the National Institute of Mental Health.

References

Chodoff, P., Friedman, S. B., and Hamburg, D. A.: Stress, defenses and coping behavior: Observations in parents of children with malignant disease, *Amer. J. Psychiat.* 120:743, 1964.

Friedman, S. B.: Care of the family of the child with cancer, *Pediat.* (Suppl.) 40:498, 1967.

Friedman, S. B.: Management of death of a parent or sibling in *Ambulatory Pediatrics,* Morris Green and Robert J. Haggerty (eds.), Philadelphia: Saunders, 1968.

Friedman, S. B., Chodoff, P., Mason, J. W., and Hamburg, D. A.: Behavioral observations in parents anticipating the death of a child. *Pediat.* 32:610, 1963.

Friedman, S. B., Karon, M., and Goldsmith, G.: Childhood leukemia: A pamphlet for parents. Dept. of Health, Education & Welfare, 1962. Revised Editions, 1965, 1967.

Friedman, S. B., Mason, J. W., and Hamburg, D. A.: Urinary 17-hydroxycorticosteroid levels in parents of children with neoplastic disease: A study of chronic psychological stress, *Psychosom. Med.* 25:364, 1963.

Karon M., and Vernick, J.: An approach to the emotional support of fatally ill children. *Clin. Ped.,* 7:274, 1968.

Lindemann, E.: Symptomatology and management of acute grief. *Am. J. Psychiat.* 101:141, 1944.

Vernick, J., and Karon, M.: Who's afraid of death on a leukemia ward? *Am. J. Dis. Child.* 109:393, 1965.

Williams, H.: On a teaching hospital's responsibility to counsel parents concerning their child's death. *Med. J. Aust.* 2:643, 1963.

PARTICIPANTS

Carmine Bedotto, M.D.
Bascom Palmer Eye Institute
University of Miami School of
  Medicine
Department of Ophthalmology
Miami, Florida

Stuart B. Brown, M.D.
Assistant Professor of Neurology
  & Pediatrics
University of Miami School of
  Medicine
Miami, Florida

C. Dean Buckner
Department of Medicine
University of Washington School
  of Medicine
U.S. Public Health Service Hospital
Seattle, Washington

Audrey E. Evans, M.D.
Associate Professor of Pediatrics
University of Pennsylvania
Director, Department of Oncology
The Children's Hospital
Philadelphia, Pennsylvania

Joseph F. Fraumeni, Jr., M.D.
Head, Ecology Studies Section
Epidemiology Branch
National Cancer Institute
Bethesda, Maryland

Arnold I. Freeman, M.D.
Department of Pediatrics
Roswell Park Memorial Institute
Buffalo, New York

Stanford B. Friedman, M.D.
Departments of Pediatrics and
  Psychiatry
University of Rochester School of
  Medicine and Dentistry
Rochester, New York

Ronald B. Herberman, M.D.
Head, Cellular and Tumor
  Immunology Section
Laboratory of Cell Biology
National Cancer Institute
Bethesda, Maryland

R. D. T. Jenkin, M.B., F.R.C.P.(C)
The Ontario Cancer Institute
The Princess Margaret Hospital
Toronto, Canada

Kjell Koch, M.D., M.S. (Peds)
Department of Pediatrics
University of Miami School of
  Medicine
Miami, Florida

August Miale, Jr., M.D.
Associate Professor of Radiology
University of Miami School of
  Medicine
Chief, Nuclear Medicine Service
Jackson Memorial Hospital
Miami, Florida

Catherine A. Poole, M.D.
Associate Professor of Radiology
  & Pediatrics
Department of Radiology
University of Miami School of
  Medicine
Miami, Florida

Lucius F. Sinks, M.D.
Department of Pediatrics
Roswell Park Memorial Institute
Buffalo, New York

J. Lawton Smith, M.D.
Professor of Ophthalmology
Professor of Neurosurgery
University of Miami School of
  Medicine
Miami, Florida

185

James L. Talbert, M.D.
Professor of Surgery and Chief
 of Pediatric Surgery
University of Florida College
 of Medicine
Coordinator of Florida Regional
 Medical Program's Children's
 Cancer Project
Gainesville, Florida

Gordon F. Vawter, M.D.
Associate Professor of Pathology
Children's Hospital Medical Center
Harvard Medical School
Associate Pathologist-in-Chief
The Children's Hospital Medical
 Center
Boston, Massachusetts

Mario M. Vuksanovic, M.D.
Clinical Professor of Radiology
University of Miami School of
 Medicine
Director, Department of
 Radiation Oncology
Cedars of Lebanon Medical Center
Miami, Florida

I. G. Williams, M.B., F.R.C.S., F.F.R.
Consultant Radiotherapist
St. Bartholomew's Hospital and
 the Hospital for Sick Children
Great Ormond Street
London, England

SUBJECT INDEX